Comfort in Birth Method™

A toolkit for mamas and doulas to achieve a calm birth

By Julie Larsen

Revised 3rd Edition 2025©

 New Reordered Edition and more content edition – Third Edition

New notes: All students should send emails to catholicdoulaprogram@gmail.com if there is another email listed in here – please email.

DEDICATION

To: Katia LeMone: She was my first midwife and my favorite.
To my husband Carl: Who is always my "cool snowman".

Letter of Introduction:

Dearest Mothers and Birth Workers.

We are glad to support you in your birth and upcoming work as a doula. We hope that this extended edition will be of service to you and that you will be able to learn more from this edition.

If you see any errors in links and such, please let us know and we will correct them in the next edition. We know the Internet is every changing!

Our goal for this course for doulas are to make you a powerful doula!

#1 A weekend training is not enough! That is why we are offering this book and as part of a full course online. You can take your time to do it or finish it fast! But you will have much more support than a weekend class!

#2 The Comfort in Birth™ Method is going to be your number one tool in your belt as a doula. Once you understand how to use this method – you will be amazed on how you can help mothers. Also, you will have clarity on what the mother's needs are – because she has filled out her enrichment form with her desires and needs – no more guess work for your next birth experience. Some mothers may not want all those "natural treatments". So, this method gives you the best way to know how to help the mother.

#3 You will not be making mistakes with our method! This method will help you know how to help mothers and anticipate their needs. Also, if you take our "Doing Business the Doula Way" Master Class – you will even learn more on how to get your business up and running. All Comfort in Birth™ method students can ask for a discount on that class!

#4 Knowing that birth is special and scientific too! Being at a birth for the first time will make you feel like you need to know so much more – so do not consider yourself an expert – however, science is also on your side of things – just observing birth can help you see the science behind things. Part of *Comfort in Birth* method is exploring and knowing science behind things – remember to look up the evidence! And remember it is OK to say – you do not know everything. A mother will understand.

#5 Do not forget to charge what you are worth as a doula. An empowered doula, you should be offering what you are worth as a doula. This will vary depending on where you are located at. Again, you will learn some things in this book and our master class. So, make sure you ask about the class too.

#6 Disclaimer: This book is not meant to replace any medical advice. This book is not meant to treat, diagnose, or prescribe anything for anyone or any mother. A mother is always in charge of her birth and desires. We support the mother's decisions during her time of labor and birth!

#7 I am always open to suggestions and additions to this manual, so please contact me if you have any questions or comments! Thank you.

Julie Larsen, author of this book!

Welcome to "Comfort in Birth™ Method" Training!
You can be an empowered doula![i]

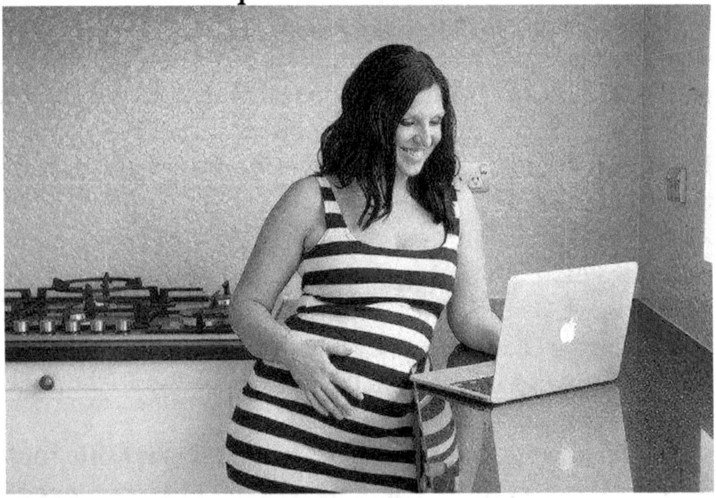

<u>Chapter One: Introduction to Birth Land![ii]</u>

Welcome, Mama or Doula! This book welcomes you to the "birth land". I hope that you will learn something from our manual for birth workers or doulas. My goal in this book is to create a manual that you can write in, take notes, and learn from. There will be blank areas in the book where you can draw and write your thoughts. This book is meant for doulas to help mamas – so we will be addressing doulas or birth workers mostly in this book and clients as mamas.

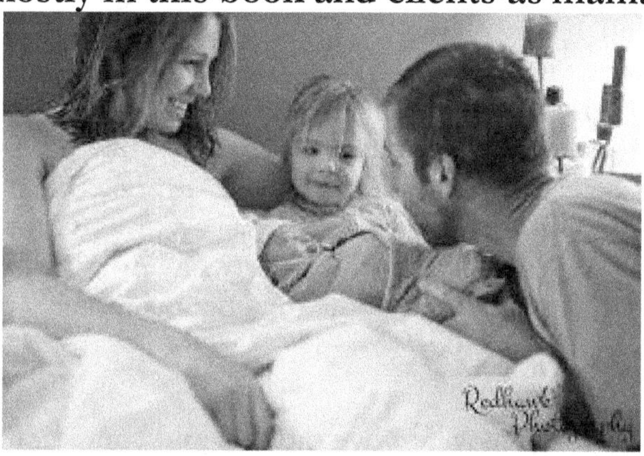

What is the "birth land?" I feel like I got into the birth world with my first child. It is a land of no return as a parent. You experience birth as a mother for the first time and this "land" is a time or place that you will never forget. I define this "birth land" as a time, place, situation that a mother experiences during her pregnancy, childbirth, or labor that she "never forgets." It is like a "moment in time" that you go back to and remember for the rest of your life.

Here is an example of one of those moments from a friend (Rosa) used with permission:

Rosa was calm as she felt her water "pop". She had been watching TV with her husband that day. "Ouch!" She exclaimed. Her husband Ralph said, "What's up?" Rosa said, "I think my water broke." As they prepared for going to the hospital, Rosa called her doctor, "The contractions are not too bad. Can we wait a bit to go?" The doctor said: "You can wait at the house for a bit but come in when they get stronger." Rosa nodded. Rosa said to Ralph, "Let me go take a shower." Ralph nodded and helped her over to the shower. Rosa said, "My back may feel better after some warm water." So, Rosa took a shower and then she decided to lay down for a bit as things seemed to calm down. Ralph prepared the hospital bags and they both went to sleep. Rosa awoke in the morning and said, "Oh, dear, I feel like I need to push." Ralph was worried, "Shall I call an ambulance?" As he was saying that he knew by the look in Rosa's eyes that it was too late for that. She pushed out their baby and he caught the "baby" in his arms. Ralph exclaimed, "It's a boy!" Rosa smiled and said, "His name is Isaac just like the Bible. He made me laugh as he came down. He is such a surprise birth!" Rosa and Ralph went later to the hospital to make sure everything was ok. Rosa said, "This is how I experienced 'birth land' by having a surprise home birth unassisted!"[iii] (Note: Quoted items may be in smaller type fonts throughout this manual).

Questions should be answered by students and emailed to comfortinbirth@gmail.com or catholicdoulanews@gmail.com

Question: If you are a mother, have you experienced "birth land" before? How did this feel to you? Write down your thoughts about "birth land" and send to instructor.

Defining a doula. A doula (Greek "servant") is a professional who is trained to be a mother's birth coach to help her with comfort, physical, and spiritual measures during pregnancy, childbirth, and postpartum time. A doula does not offer any medical advice or do any medical procedures. A birth doula offers continuous care that is vital for pregnancy and labor. A birth doula spends at least 10 hours or more with her client (mother) in order to gain confidence before the birth. A birth doula does not displace the father/partner or dad. The birth doula helps the father gain confidence at birth and suggests ways he can help the mother.

Question: How do you define a doula? What does a doula do?

<u>Defining comfort in birth. Comfort in Birth Method™</u>

This means the mother is relaxed, comfortable, breathes well, has rhythm, understand baby positioning and births in a way that is less painful (when possible, all natural) way during her "birth time." Part of this method is creating the sacred space for birth as well as understanding certain techniques for labor. In other words, the mother enjoys "comfort in birth" through her own experience or journey and this can vary depending on the mother's choices at birth! Note: We will go over more about "Comfort in Birth" later.

What if a mother wants an epidural just because? Does this mean this is not part of the method? No, we feel that a mother needs to find her comfort zone for labor. If this means, she obtains an epidural for laboring then that is great. This is still a "comfort in birth" for this mother! So, Comfort in Birth Method™ can have various meaning for each mother. Our goal is to present the relaxation and techniques to help a mother achieve the best birth possible outcome. A comfort in birth can be all natural and have little pain with the help of a doula or comfort techniques. The focus of this booklet is to help the mother achieve the best natural birth. We will explain a little more about Comfort in Birth later as well. *Disclaimer: We are not attempting or will ever offer any diagnosis – this is up to a doctor or other medical practitioner to determine if a mother needs certain drugs, medications, or advice.*

Question: How would you define "comfort in birth"? Write this in your own words.

Define rebozo. A rebozo is a Mexican[iv] shawl (other countries make them) that a mother can use as a tool for her upcoming birth. A rebozo can also be used to carry the baby in after birth depending on the size. Doulas will usually learn how to offer these comfort techniques to the mother. Rebozo is also a key tool for our "comfort in birth" philosophy! We will be presenting a couple of techniques in this manual. Students are welcome to

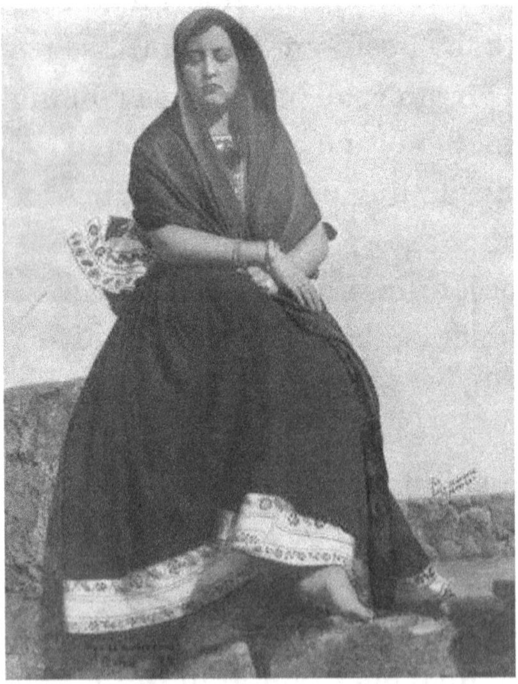

take as an extra class "Royal Rebozo Way" Course levels from us – message instructor for details.

~~~~~~~~Mexican Rebozo Expanded Section~~~~~

"The Mexican rebozo originated in colonial times and is a piece of clothing extensively used by Mexican women today. The rebozo is square linen that is used to cover the upper body and head. It is used to carry babies in traditional Mexico, and more recently around the world. It is also a luxury garment used for special celebrations.

In history, Fray Diego Duran mentions them for the first time in the XVI century saying that rebozos were knitted in Oaxaca with cotton and silk. To this elegant garment, knitters would add metallic threads and other ornaments to make a luxury complement for affluent women of the time.

The rebozo is a part of Mexican history. In 1757 there was a law that legislated over the size, knitting, thread class and design. Following Roman Catholic traditions, the Virgin of Angustias was named the saint to advocate for the knitters of rebozos: las rebozeras."[v]

Origin of the Mexican Rebozo[vi] – according to online source:

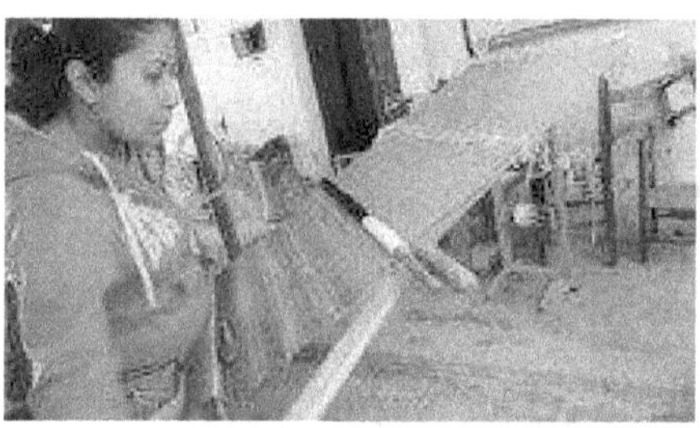

"The most traditional Mexican rebozos used to be from Sultepec in today's State of Mexico knitted with a waist loom as early as 1573 when Diego Cortes Chimalpopoca was Cacique of the region.

In Puebla, you can find the famous golden rebozos of taffeta, which is silk, weave with a specific pattern of threads.

In Saltillo, you can find the traditional "saw teeth" design which is the same style used in Mexican Serapes.

Classical rebozos are made out of cotton and silk. They are decorated using a technique called marbling (jaspeado in Spanish). This old fashion way of dyeing consists of making knots in sections of the threads so that the color does not impregnate consistently. The technique gives a beautiful irregular marbling or stripe appearance exposing the tint and the natural color of the fiber. After the knitting, the threads from the side are tied making a nice design or maybe a phrase.

Today's elegant Mexican rebozos are knitted by:

- The Matlatzincas from Tenancingo in the State of Mexico.
- The Purepechas from La Piedad, Zamora and Tanganicuaro in the State of Michoacan.
- The Nahuas from Chilapa in the State of Guerrero, and
- The Otomis from Santa Maria del Rio in the State of San Luis Potosi.

In 1951, in Santa Maria del Rio, it was founded the school of rebozo knitting to maintain the tradition that was disappearing. They master the marbling or jaspeado technique, and create authentic pieces of art. For example, the one-color silk rebozo with amazing beauty and elegance."[vii]

We will talk more about the "rebozo" in another chapter.

What does a doula do?

*She offers prenatal Education: though this should be limited for a doula to offer – if a mother needs more of a fuller childbirth class series – she should either a) signup with one with you if you have credentials to teach or b) encourage her to find an online or local class to take.

*She offers: Birth Plan, "Birth Wishes" or "Birth Vision": A doula needs to understand how to make a birth plan up to help parents. Some seasoned parents will not need this as much – if so then have them consider another type of preparatory class like learning about the rebozo.

*She offers: Birth Preparation: A doula usually helps with birth preparation in the way that she shows the parents what she is going to offer during labor. She will go over comfort measures and techniques that you learn later on in this booklet. Also, we always encourage doulas that train with us that it is okay to take another doula training. If you want to learn more from another organization, we have no problem with that! We know all organizations have various things to learn. So, feel free to share our information as long as a person knows it is copyrighted.

*She offers releasing fears of birth: We can show you some tips on helping moms release fears as part of being a doula. Many moms have birth fears, and this is normal. If their fears seem to take over their life, then that is abnormal, and they may want to seek a doctor's help for prenatal anxiety or prenatal depression. *Ask us for Letting go of fears separate sheet to go through with a mother.

*She offers: Home Visits – 2 prenatal, 1 postpartum: Now that we are in "covid" times – the "home visits" may take place via zoom with a client to be. You may only be going up to the hospital when the time comes if the hospital allows doulas. Many hospitals are now allowing doulas – but you will need to follow their protocols (wearing a mask, being tested, maybe even wearing certain clothes) and that may mean getting a "covid" test that might not be accurate. So, if it comes out "positive" demand a retest as some of those tests are not that accurate; make sure you know your rights as well as the patient knowing their rights. Have the hospital staff "literally read aloud" the patient bill of rights to your client esp. if the client has specific needs. You may want to do is get tested by a private doctor vs. hospital so that you can just have the results before going up to the hospital. If a hospital does not require testing, then that is great. It may depend on the hospital. Postpartum visit can also be done via zoom if the parents do not wish to have you near them after the baby's birth. Respect whatever decisions they make. It is not your baby. If they want you to visit with masks and gloves on, then please respect that. Working with clients during these times is very trying for everyone; remember to keep a positive attitude. Being aware of universal precautions is important too.

*She helps with Optimal Fetal Positioning – best position for baby's birth:

We also recommend you go to Spinning Babies website to learn more about optimal fetal positioning. www.spinningbabies.com – The Belly Mapping book we recommend for a book review plus you get to learn something fun: https://www.spinningbabies.com/product/belly-mapping-workbook/

*She helps with Rebozo techniques: We offer a fuller class you can take separately – please ask instructor for special pricing deal for being a "Comfort in Birth Method™ student." There will be a few techniques in this book.

*She helps with Birth Story: Sharing the mother's birth story – writing it down is important. What does she want to share?

A doula can help with Belly Binding: This is usually done after mother has had her baby – so mostly a postpartum doula technique, but any doula can learn. Binding the belly helps the mothers' organs move back into place after birth.

A doula is not a midwife; so, she does not offer any medical side of things and cannot take blood pressure, measure the fundus, etc. However, if a mother wants to learn how to do this on her own, she should be encouraged to do so. A mother can even learn how to do her own urine samples! We always think a mother should take charge of her own health!

Explore More! This section of the book – sometimes you will explore a website or there maybe an assignment attached to explore more. For this section, please look over the websites below.

DONA International: www.dona.org

First doula organization

Evidence Based Birth: www.evidencebasedbirth.com "Evidence for doulas"

Inspired Birth Pro: www.inspiredbirthpro.com

CAPPA: www.cappa.net

Childbirth International: https://childbirthinternational.com/birth-doula/ Think of other doula organizations you might want to look up or resource websites that help mothers:

https://pcoschallenge.org/ , https://ndss.org/ , https://americanpregnancy.org/ , https://www.elizabethhouse.net/

Questions:

Are there any birth philosophies listed? What is the mission statement if listed? Submit to instructor.

Write down your own goals for your current doula training. What do you wish to accomplish? When do you want to finish? Send it to instructor.

CHAPTER 2: HISTORY OF CHILDBIRTH & DOULAS PLUS WHAT IS A MIDWIFE

Birth is as old as history itself. Biblical times to now; we have birthed without doctors longer than having doctors' help. Let us look at the history of birth from around 1600 to the present day. ***The history of birth is a fascinating subject.***

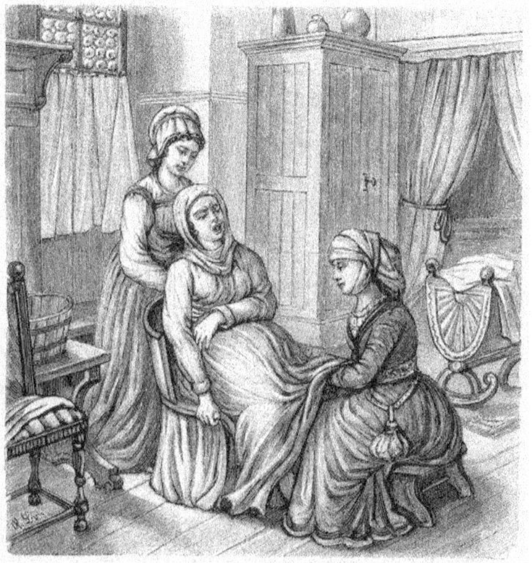

1600's: The Royal birth was "attended" by many people in the room. Thus, the Queen was basically stressed out with her labor being watched by so many people. This was done for various reasons – one to make sure that a girl was not switched for a boy. However, in the instance of this article I found, the Queen of France had a boy named Louis France![viii]

1700's: Our history timeline begins mid-1700's – the forceps were developed which helped with deliveries that were considered difficult.[ix]

Granny midwifery began in our country with arrival of African slaves (so around the time of the civil war era and beyond.) They practiced up until around the 1940's when most of them were ousted because they were not "medical doctors" and hand no training like midwifery

schooling. Granny midwives delivered up to 75 percent of the babies in the southwest regions up to around the 1940's or so.[x]

1800's chloroform was used during childbirth deliveries. Another remedy to help during delivery was a mixture of alcohol and oatmeal in a drink. So, you might say women drank "birth beer" during labor! It also helped with healing during postpartum time frame.[xi] Sometimes women during childbirth would cook a cake during labor – this cake was called a "groaning cake." This at least kept women more upright during labor and moving around. I could imagine doing this if in early labor. I might need help if I was in deeper active labor, that cake better be in the oven by then![xii]

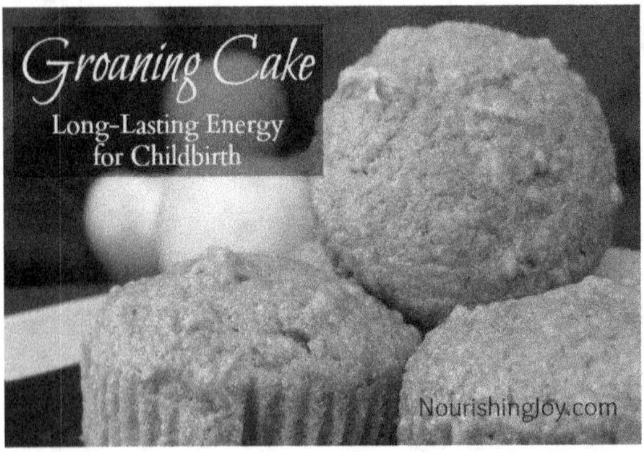

Midwives attended births way before men ever came on the scene. So, midwifery was common up to around the 1800's. Men started taking over birth pretty quickly. Hospitals when established preferred to have men as doctors.

In the 18th to 19th centuries, women died of "puerperal fever" during childbirth because they did not understand the need for cleanliness at childbirth. A doctor working with the dead would then go deliver a baby! So, many women died during childbirth that they had wills made out before they went into labor. The reason for this "fever" is that the doctors did not wash their hands between handling women and then handling dead bodies. Quite shocking![xiii]

Routine handwashing and such did not really become a practice until around 1875, despite a doctor that suggested this needed to be done earlier than that. Also, instruments were also sterilized at around the same time. I imagine you could sterilize them by putting them in a hot stove or heat. Nowadays, I am sure there is chemicals and sterilization techniques.

Early 1900's (specifically around 1914), Twilight sleep was a way of childbirth in Germany (and spread to other countries) where women were drugged with morphine and scopolamine during childbirth, and they woke up with no memory of the birth or what happened. The women would become violent because of the drug, so they were basically tied down to the beds and the doctors would deliver the baby without the mother recalling being tied down and such. Anyway, there is more to this story that we do not have time to share all of this. Research "Twilight Sleep" on your own if you want to learn more. One thing to note – twilight sleep did not take away the pain of labor even though it was called "painless childbirth" by the Germans. The drug that was used to block memory also helped block the mother's memory of being in pain during labor! This movement spread from Germany to USA around 1914 or so. This movement stayed pretty much in USA through the 1960's.[xiv]

In the early 1970's Twilight sleep *was not used for birth anymore*. In fact, my mom remembers giving birth at the hospital and she didn't want any drugs at my birth, but the doctors gave her something where she couldn't see anything- like she blacked out – but she could still hear what was going on. So, she was a bit drugged in a different way when I was born! Anyway, the birth movement started being more natural minded around this time.

Let us back up a little bit and talk about breastfeeding as this is a part of our history as well.

Breastfeeding was at an all-time low in the 1950's, so Mary White and Marian Thompson founded La Leche League in 1956. This organization is now worldwide. However, the ideas of the organization have changed over time and is more liberal in their beliefs than what the original founders had formed.[xv]

In 1969, Dana Raphael coined the term "doula" to the world. Now, the word doula means "servant or slave" in Greek. This term sticks today to define doulas all over who help mothers in labor, but do not offer medical services!

Born in 1930, Michael Odent is still alive at the time of this writing. He is a physician and obstetrician that worked with women awhile back in France. He basically introduced the idea of homebirth in hospital. His hospital was set up much like a home birthing room or like today's birth centers. The mothers that came to birth there were more educated by him and his staff. Michael Odent believed that babies should have a nice warm bath right after birth and would encourage mothers to give their babies this special bath. Michael wrote "Birth Reborn" and other books about birth. He also had a special clinic to help mothers have more natural births.

Biddy Mason was a "slave" in Georgia and was given as a gift to someone for their "wedding gift." Now, she was someone else's slave. Her owners were Mormons, so they traveled around for the Mormon Church. We can assume that was probably around Utah area. They were going to settle in California (around 1851); however, they had just passed laws freeing slaves there. So, the owners wanted to move down to Texas. Miss Biddy Mason made her escape and became a free slave and became a nurse midwife in the Los Angeles area. Onnie Lee Logan is another famous midwife from Alabama, and she was African American. She managed to become a midwife as well and delivered lots of babies. She has a biography book. Margaret Charles Smith is considered one of the last "Granny" midwives. She went to midwifery school in 1949. Most of her clients were poor and malnourished. She delivered thousands of babies. You may want to read her biography: *"The Life Story of Alabama Midwife."*[xvi]

Extra reading: https://blackmidwivesalliance.org/legacy-1/f/what-is-the-legacy-of-black-midwives-in-the-us-and-caribbean

Ina May Gaskin started the Farm midwives in the 1970's and offered natural childbirth options to mothers. Many mothers would travel to Tennessee just to birth with a "farm midwife" in order to experience more natural birth. Ina May Gaskin also wrote a book "Spiritual Midwifery" which is still read today as one of the most popular books. The Farm Midwives do still exist, and they do offer in person classes if someone is interested in learning more go to: http://thefarmmidwives.org/

DONA International was founded in the 1990's and started training doulas through their organization. www.dona.org

Catholic Doula Program started in 2014 to train doulas in a more Catholic way. The program includes birth, postpartum, and bereavement doula training. www.catholicdoula.com

Question: Name three things you learned about the history of childbirth? What would you like to explore more?

Timeline History Enrichment Activity A: This is like an assignment for doulas in training to do if taking for our class. Otherwise you can also do for fun.

Write up your own timeline history of childbirth. What would it look like? You can start with a certain time frame like 1800 to the present day.

The second part of your timeline can be your own added timeline, have you experienced birth, what things are important to you as far as becoming a doula? When did you first learn about doula work? Include things like that in the second part if you choose to add that to the timeline.

What is a midwife? A midwife means "with woman".[xvii]

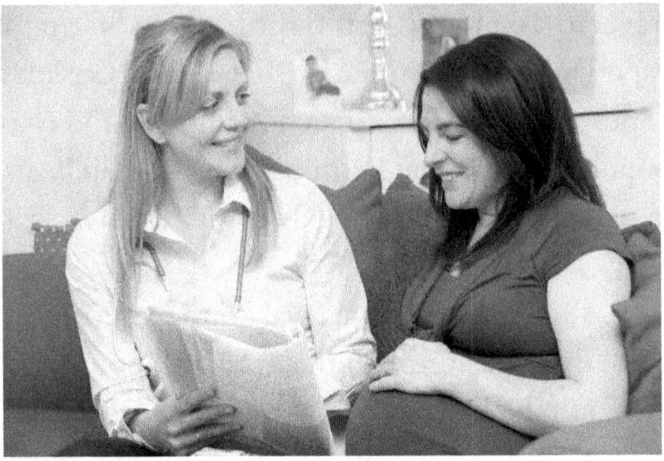

A midwife prepares a mother for birth and assists at the delivery of the baby when it is time for labor. The midwife does not usually offer drugs or epidurals to a mother seeking a natural delivery. The midwife only offers the most natural birth possible. Some midwives can also act as doulas or "monitrice". A monitrice is someone who can offer more medical side of things (like cervical checks) but then works with the doctor or hospital to get the mother to the hospital in timely manner. A monitrice also may assist a midwife as well.

A midwife does:

Blood pressure checks
Urinal analysis
Palpitations of the uterus
Leopold's maneuvers
Optimal fetal positioning
Cervical checks
Pap smear (usually after birth or before pregnancy)
Hemoglobin checks
Blood tests

IV's for fluids (possibly antibiotics if she is working under a doctor)

Oxygen

Neonatal Resuscitation

Pitocin – synthetic – this is only if she has permission in her state to do so.

Other ways to stop bleeding after birth such as herbs, homeopathy, etc.

Note: In each chapter we will have discussion questions for you to do for credit if taking this as a doula student. (Otherwise no need to do). Some chapters will have quizzes too.

Question: What is a doula?

Question: What is a midwife? What does she do?

Question: Who coined the word doula? (Hint: In history section).

Question: What is a monitrice?

Terms – We ask you to make a definition list of around 50-60 doula terms. So, the above questions will get you started on that list!

Enrichment B: What is the evidence for doulas? What does this mean? Evidence for doulas means we are looking for statistics on how hiring a doula can reduce the rate or scale of mother getting into trouble during labor. Did the doula help reduce something? What? www.evidencebasedbirth.com is one site you can go to for this information.

***Submit your "evidence of doula" assignment to catholicdoulanews@gmail.com or comfortinbirth@gmail.com – you may also combine it with above "What is a doula?" and make a beautiful doula brochure for your clients!

CHAPTER 3: Comfort in Birth plus Emotions of Labor.

Comfort in Birth Acronym meaning and our philosophy:

C means Calm = Achieving a Calming atmosphere for birth and a sacred space for birth. C also means ***Comfort in birth*** of course! What is comfortable for the mother at this period of time in her birth time? A birth free of pain as much as possible. This is our goal.

O means Oxytocin = O means Oxytocin =

What is Oxytocin? "Oxytocin is released through various stimuli, including physical touch, social bonding, and childbirth, promoting feelings of love and trust."[xviii] - source: https://wellwisp.com/how-is-oxytocin-released/

Quoted article: **"Oxytocin is often dubbed the "love hormone," a title that speaks volumes about its role in human relationships. This fascinating peptide hormone plays a significant role in social bonding, emotional regulation, and even childbirth. Understanding how oxytocin is released can shed light on its profound effects on our emotional and physical well-being.**

The Biological Mechanism of Oxytocin Release

The release of oxytocin primarily occurs in the hypothalamus, a small region at the base of the brain. From there, it travels through the posterior pituitary gland into the bloodstream. This process can be triggered by various factors, including physical touch, emotional connections, and certain physiological events.

Oxytocin release isn't just a simple switch that gets flipped; it involves complex interactions between various neurotransmitters and hormones. For instance, during childbirth, the stretching of the cervix and uterus sends signals to the brain to release oxytocin. This release not only aids in labor but also fosters maternal bonding right after birth.

Research has shown that oxytocin levels rise during intimate activities such as hugging or cuddling. The warmth of another person's touch can stimulate sensory neurons that send signals to the brain to release this powerful hormone. The act of breastfeeding also triggers oxytocin release in mothers, reinforcing the emotional bond between mother and child.

Factors Influencing Oxytocin Release

Several factors influence how oxytocin is released in our bodies. These factors range from biological triggers to environmental cues.

1. Physical Touch

Physical contact plays a crucial role in stimulating oxytocin release. Activities like hugging, kissing, or even simple hand-holding can significantly increase levels of this hormone. Studies have shown that couples who engage in regular affectionate touch report higher satisfaction in their relationships.

2. Social Interactions

Social bonding is another significant factor influencing oxytocin levels. Engaging with friends or family members fosters feelings of safety and trust, leading to increased oxytocin production. This hormonal surge not only enhances interpersonal relationships but also contributes to overall mental health.

3. Childbirth and Breastfeeding

As mentioned earlier, childbirth is a critical moment for oxytocin release. The hormone not only helps facilitate labor but also promotes maternal behaviors immediately following birth. Breastfeeding further stimulates its release as mothers bond with their infants during feeding sessions.

4. Emotional Connections

Emotional experiences can trigger oxytocin release as well. Moments of vulnerability or shared joy with loved ones can lead to increased levels of this hormone. Engaging in meaningful conversations or sharing experiences creates an emotional connection that boosts oxytocin production.

The Role of Oxytocin in Human Relationships

Oxytocin's influence extends beyond mere biological processes; it plays a pivotal role in shaping human relationships and social dynamics.

1. Enhancing Trust

One of oxytocin's most fascinating effects is its ability to enhance trust among individuals. Research has shown that higher levels of this hormone are linked to increased trustworthiness and reduced fear responses during social interactions.

This phenomenon has profound implications for building healthy relationships—whether romantic or platonic—as it encourages open communication and vulnerability among partners.

2. Strengthening Bonds

Oxytocin fosters emotional connections between individuals by promoting feelings of attachment and affection. This bond is particularly evident in parent-child relationships but extends to friendships and romantic partnerships as well.

When people engage in activities that promote oxytocin release—like spending quality time together or engaging in physical affection—they're likely to strengthen their emotional bonds over time.

3. Reducing Stress

Interestingly enough, oxytocin also plays a role in reducing stress levels within relationships. When individuals experience high stress, their bodies produce cortisol—the stress

hormone—which can negatively impact interpersonal dynamics.

However, elevated oxytocin levels counteract cortisol's effects by promoting relaxation and calmness during stressful situations. This balance allows individuals to navigate challenges together more effectively. (End of Quoted article-source[xix]

I think that is all I need to quote from this article.

Your couples you work with - we want you to encourage husband and wife to work together during childbirth and this Oxytocin will happen naturally without anything else needed.

I do mention a rebozo technique called Shake the Apples: https://www.youtube.com/watch?v=SL1qf5Uzu8Q

This rebozo technique can help **destress and help oxytocin** levels in a **natural way** but if a mother does not want this technique - then please respect her wishes.

Some rebozo people will call this "Shaking Apple Trees" as "sexual stimulation" but I think they are just meaning - this might help **raise oxytocin levels** - not meaning to have sex or anything related to anything sinful. **As Christians we are not supporting anything sinful in this class. Thank you.**

M means meditation/muscle/movement/mother = First of all meditation is a way to get mother to relax. Second using muscles (uterus) during "surges" (contractions) helps the baby move down. Third movement, as the labor progresses movement of the mother in an upright position will help the baby move down further. Movement can be various positions, using a birth ball, etc. Finally, when baby is born, a "mother is born" as well. Now, the pregnant woman is a "mother."

F means Feelings and Fears = We should acknowledge the mother's feelings and any fears she has of birth. We should help her practice fear releasing techniques and calm meditation in order to overcome these fears or feelings.

O means open = Opening the body to birth. O can also be for Options for birth. Has the mother chosen the right options for her birth? This is her choice. Remember to be an advocate for her choices not yours.

R means Relaxation = We teach relaxation techniques such as breathing, using rebozo, and meditation.

T means Tools and Techniques and Touch =

Tools such as rebozo, massage, acupressure, the healing arts are important for a mother to know about. Trusting the birth process is important. Explore the website www.trustinbirth.com

Touch is another important aspect of our method. ***Touching the mother during labor should be done with her permission, gently*** (when you can), or at least done in a "modest" way – meaning doing it in a way that will help the mother be comfortable. (This can be for either "T" in the acronym). We will explain a little more about touch in our rebozo booklet – so please make sure you receive that if taking the full course!

B means Buoyancy, Breathe, Baby = First of all buoyancy of water – if a mother decides on a water birth the rules seem to change a bit. How do I explain this? I had a water birth with my third child. It was amazing experience. One minute I was feeling a lot of pain in my back (I had also been in a car wreck a couple of days earlier) and then when I got into the water tub almost all pain melted away. It was the best therapy for birth I could have ever wanted.

Second, B for baby. Continuing my story of water birth. I was able to breathe (another "b") out my baby by using a "blowing" technique. I would "blow" during my time off from the surges and then breathe with the surge. I was able to "blow" and "bring" my baby down to me and he was "born". It was just an awesome experience. He was born in the water. So, Water (buoyancy), *Breathing and Baby are important steps together.*

I means "I can" do it! I can give birth! Ignite this in the mother if she is feeling the mode of "I cannot do this." This is important emotional support which we cover more below!

R means Rhythm and Ritual. We already mentioned relaxation above. *Rhythm is getting into a rhythm during childbirth and delivery.* Usually for me this happens around transition to pushing baby out. *Other mothers may find a rhythm earlier on.* It also depends upon the birth. Finding the right rhythm is important to feeling more relaxed and having a "comfort" birth. *Ritual is another thing to explore for each mother from whatever culture she is from.*

T means Time. Birth takes time. There should not be a rushing it idea. A mother should have the right to take the time she needs. This is why if going to hospital to wait as long as possible unless you have a reason to go in earlier.

H means Healing. We believe Comfort in Birth Method© will be a healing experience for many mothers. Offering her an alternative to a previous C-section or previous traumatic birth. We hope that offering this Comfort in Birth Method© will allow healing process to occur.

Now that you understand the **Comfort in Birth Method© ideals or process.** Let us try a case study below to apply our method. A case study is a type of story that helps you think, and you may also research topics that are important too. In this case study, *we are exploring pain theory.*

Grantly Dick-Read came up with the pain theory the idea of *"fear = tension = pain".* Well, today you may see that even more outside of the birth realm. However, we will keep on topic.

So, if a mother has fears of delivery and pain, then she will tense up more and then she will feel pain more. That's the basis of the theory.

So, what remedies can we offer women who get into this cycle of fear-tension-pain? Can they still achieve a calm birth experience and a "comfort" birth? Yes, if you can work with a mother in early labor and or before birth process begins. Some of this is a mindset while for other mothers it is more than that. Each mother perceives pain differently. Some mothers may have a lot of trouble handling pain. In that case, we suggest she uses an epidural and still attempt the birth with the rest of the Comfort in Birth techniques. It is okay if a mom wants an epidural at her birth. Our method is not just about natural birth; it is about the mom wants to have at her birth. Honoring her wishes is the highest form of humility as a doula.

We will cover more about pain in our pain chapter.

Handout Resources go here to see a full library from Penny Simkin: https://www.pennysimkin.com/articles-resources/ **- We may send you something from this library to look over.**

What is a Case Study? A case study is something made up or real that you will study and learn from. You may be asked to do more research after reading the case study. Here is your first one below:

Case Study: Isabelle is a Jewish girl, and she is attached to her family; but her husband is not allowed at the birth according to Jewish customs. So, Isabelle must only birth with other women in her family. However, Isabelle's mother-in-law wants to come and Isabelle does not like her that much. (problem one). Second, Isabelle has a lot of fear about pain in labor and needs some assurance and techniques to help her out (second problem). Third, Isabelle is very shy about modesty during delivery – she would like to be covered up as much as possible, but still have some freedom of movement at the birth center (This particular birth center may only allow limited movement). (Third issue). Find remedies or ideas for Isabelle's three issues listed. Also, consider the Comfort in Birth Method© as mentioned above for this case study. Consider tools that might be handy for a birth that is readily available (birth ball, rebozo, massage tool, etc.) *Please answer the 3 questions – use separate paper and turn into instructor.*

A more spiritual application of the ***Word "CALM" acronym #2.***

Now, if you feel this section is not for you – please skip to the next one about emotions and childbirth. However, if you want a deeper spiritual meaning – please read. In my doula practice, I am a Catholic Doula, so some of this may not pertain to your religion; however, I hope you will bear with me and just get the "understanding" of the practice here. You may use your own words for the acronym if so desired.

C = Christ. Jesus Christ is my Savior. He is the One I lean on during prayer. I feel a Calm inside my soul when I surrender my will to Jesus. So, this C can also mean Calm, Centered, or even surrender. This means we are asking Jesus (or your belief) to enter in and help you establish a connection to Him during this pregnancy or to your mama client.

A = Allow. Allow means allowing God, Christ, Jesus, or (name your belief) to work within you. This allowing process helps especially when a mother is scared or uncertain about her pregnancy or birth. Allow is also another step-in surrender (above). We are allowing God to work within our souls and hearts. As a birth worker, you are allowing Him to enter into your actions. So, A can stand for Actions. Are you offering worthy actions?

L = Learn and Leads Us. God teaches us about Himself everyday through His word the Bible. God leads us to a deeper meaning of childbirth and pregnancy. We also as birth workers are learning the process of birth and asking God to lead us to a better understanding of the birth process and His love for us. Learn and Lead also mean that sometimes birth does not result in what we wanted or expected. Sometimes there is sorrow or pain while other times there is a mini miracle during that mother's delivery!

M = Mother or meditation. I know some of you reading this are not Catholic or Christian. So, "M" can stand for a Meditative state. Mother is a good one to consider. We all have mothers and we are also becoming a Mother during childbirth and labor. So, this is the best word for anyone to consider we are becoming a mother at birth. If one is Catholic, they can consider *Mother Mary as a patroness of their childbirth and labor. Mary had Jesus in her womb, so we can think about this as a meditation too.*

Meditation: This is a way to enter into childbirth in a more spiritual way. Some may call it hypnosis. It is a way to enter deeper into the birth and accept the process of birthing. Meditation for me includes images in my mind of Jesus, Mother Mary, or the Apostles of Christ during Jesus' life. Like meditation on the Life and death of Jesus Christ. If you are another spirituality, then you will probably have your own method of meditation.

Question: Now that you have a better understanding of the acronym "Comfort in Birth" – re-define your earlier definition of this method – what does it mean to you?

Question: Define CALM in your own words. How would you use either acronym (Comfort in birth or calm) for helping a mother during her pregnancy or childbirth?[xx]

Emotions and childbirth method:

Now we will cover the emotions of childbirth and labor. We kind of "borrow" these ideas from the *Bradley method*, though I do not know the full extent of this method. The emotions at childbirth and labor are very defined and I noticed most of these emotions during all my labors though they varied from each child. I also notice these emotions working with mothers as a doula.

First Emotion of Childbirth: Excitement Stage:

This is usually early labor.

The mother is excited that she feels surges starting up

The mother has:

A. Initial contractions
B. Her water broke with contractions or surges.
C. She feels excited about the baby coming down.
D. She may also feel a bit nervous. If a mom calls you up in early labor – remind her to breathe and relax.

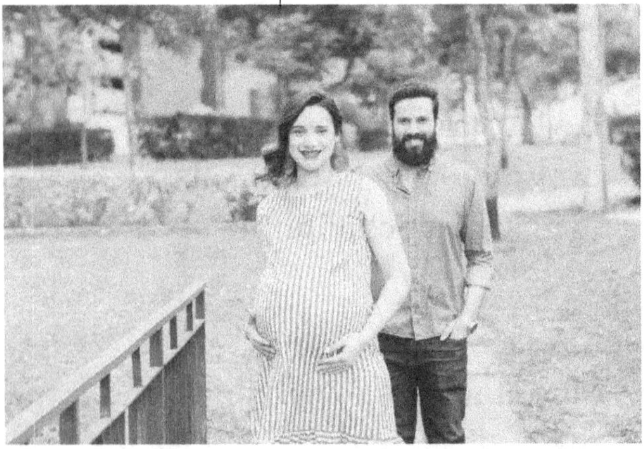

<u>Excitement – First Stage of Emotions:</u>

The mother is excited that her "time" has come. She usually can-do everyday tasks at this stage, but she is also pre-paring to get to hospital as soon as things pick up on labor. She may stay home and prepare a meal or go for a walk. *(Picture: Felipe Salgado @ unsplash.com)*

If her water broke, she may want to put on a maxi pad or something to help with the water leakage. She should call her doctor or midwife to know what to do about staying at home or heading to hospital if water breaks. If having a home birth, the midwife may come over to check mother.

Doula work: The doula most likely will be in phone contact with mother during the excitement stage or heading over to the mom's house depending on the arrangement before birth.

Second Emotion of Childbirth: Getting a bit serious or concentration stage.

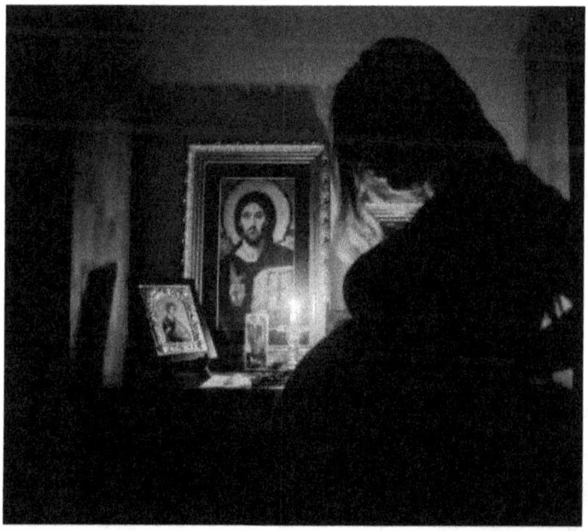

The contractions or surges are coming regularly; this is usually the time for mother to head to hospital or follow the 4-1-1 or 5-1-1 rule. (She may wait at home for a bit if earlier in this stage.)

This is usually when labor starts to hit around 4-5 centimeters. As a doula, we will not be able to check the cervix. However, the mother's voice will usually give her away. She starts having trouble talking with you. She has to concentrate more on the surges (contractions). This second emotion may last awhile depending on the length of labor. So, she may still be able to talk with you at the beginning of the serious stage and it gradually gets harder for the mother to talk with you. Towards the end of this stage if she is choosing a hospital birth, she may want to get headed over that way.

Doula work: This stage the mom may feel emotionally like a bit of a roller coaster.

As a doula, may hold the mother's hand, encourage her to breathe through the contractions/surges. Endnote picture[xxi]

Start practicing comfort measures once you arrive and get settled at hospital either in Triage or the real room. Triage is not that fun; so, make sure mom can get quickly into a room. Advocate for her to get quickly into a room if triage is necessary. Or ask if she can go straight to a room and skip triage. I had one time where they had me in some side-room as I guess since I had a tear from my home birth – I had to wait what seemed like hours to get into a room. It was very uncomfortable. It probably wasn't that long, but when a mother is in pain or not feeling well – doctors should take time to make sure she is taken care of better.

Third Emotion of Childbirth: Transition – "I cannot do this anymore."

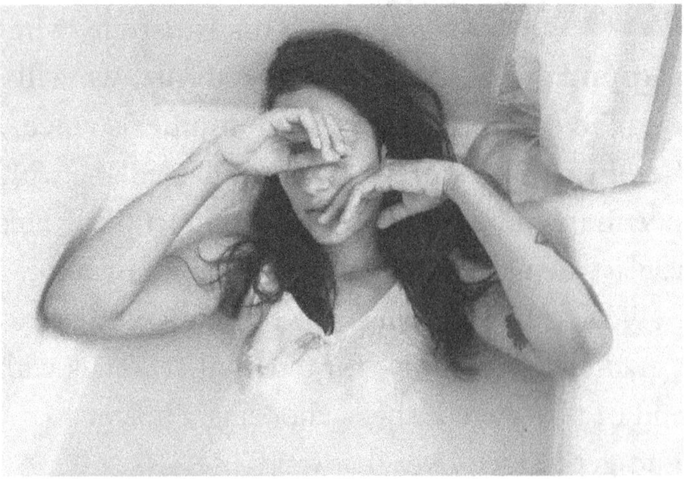

Picture: Naomi August @ unsplash.com

Transition emotions: There is usually a moment in time it may last just like a flash or longer for some mothers. It is that moment in labor where the mother just feels that she cannot go on. It happens at different time points but usually it is like transition or pushing stage of delivery. Your mom may say "I want an epidural" when she wasn't planning one or "I can't do this." She may even make a lot of noise or scream out. This emotion will usually pop up around transition stage; however, some moms have a calm transition, and it is more at the beginning of pushing stage. So, remember this emotion pops up at different times.

For instance, my home birth I think I had experienced a more calming transition, I was having some back pain, so I took the TENS unit and focused on breathing through contractions (surges) and just doing that in my own space. I probably did not realize how much time had passed. All of a sudden, I needed to "go to the bathroom". I thought I could not go on in labor. However, my midwife checked me, and I was at the pushing stage! I felt encouragement hearing this and was able to continue on and push out our baby. So, anyway, this stage of "cannot go on" happens usually around this transition or time to push. Some moms may need extra help at this time; so, it really depends on the mother.

What a doula can do for this emotional stage: You are there to support this mother emotionally. First of all, try to get **her to relax.** Tell a joke (if this mother likes that kind of thing). Or **rub her back.** Do something to make her know you are there for her. **Tell her "You can do this." She needs that**

encouragement. "You rock." Words of affirmation from Love Languages really helps right at this point of labor. If you are not familiar with the 5 love languages, we suggest you look up: www.5lovelanguages.com

One of the love language is "touch" (we talk about briefly more below) **and if a mother likes touch (you should ask her before the birth), then practicing light touch, gently stroking her arms or legs during labor, can help this "touch" mom feel better. So, remember to add touch in if the mother is getting really emotionally – it can help her calm down and center back into the stages of labor and birth**. (Note: Gentle stroking technique is also called "havening"). **However, not all mothers like touch – so remember to ask permission first before touching a mother.**

Fourth Emotion: "I did it!"

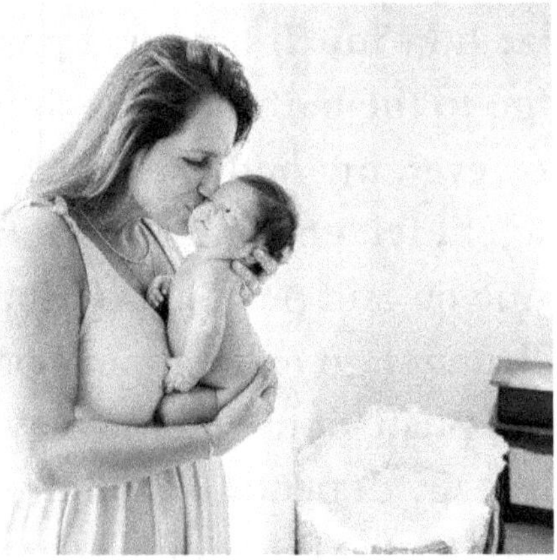

Picture Jonathan Borba @ unsplash.com

This last emotion usually happens after the mother pushes the baby out. However, encouraging the mother during her pushing saying, "you are doing a great job" will help her achieve the final goal of holding that baby and saying, "I did it!" She will rock that birth better if she has knowledge of the emotions of childbirth. **Doulas will help moms rock that labor better by being the support she needs at birth.**

A doula does is rejoice with this mother; her baby is out and in the world! Yeah, you rocked this birth! Congratulate her on this accomplishment![xxii]

Question: What are the four emotions of labor? If you are a mother, have you ever experienced any of these?

1. Emotion #1
2. Emotion #2
3. Emotion #3
4. Emotion #4

<u>The Five Love Languages – Brief Overview:</u>

The Five love languages come from a book under that title. The main summary of these are: Words of Affirmations, Touch/Hugs, Gifts, Acts of Service, Quality time.

Explore More: Look up Five Love Languages on the Internet.

www.fivelovelanguages.com

Find out – what is your love language?

If you have a doula client – what is her love language?

How can knowing a client's love language help you help her during labor? If you know your client's love language, then you can help facilitate a better understanding of her needs during labor. There are some mothers who love touch and hugs while others do not. There are some mothers who love

having the words of affirmation during labor while other mothers do not like to talk a lot. There are some mothers who love gifts (even though it is a bit hard to give gifts every minute) – but your presence at her birth is a gift for instance. You can always make her a baby gift when her baby is born! Acts of Service type of mother will love all the little things you do as a doula because it is a complete act of service to her. Last but not least is quality time – spending the right quality time with the mother is helpful for her before her baby is born – attention to details at your prenatals for instance!

Affirmations can help with the emotional and spiritual side of a "comfort in birth". We need to conclude this section by showing you some affirmation methods that can help mothers during their labors.

As a Christian doula, I like to take Scripture quotes and quotes from saints to give to mothers as part of their birth experience.

Examples: "Jesus I trust in Thee." "I breathe out my baby beautifully." "I am confident in my body's ability to give birth." "Jesus helps me breathe out my baby." "You are wonderfully made."

Affirmations can be anything the mother likes to read. If she enjoys a certain author or "guru" then affirmations can be made from this mother's favorite quotes. So, consider what the mother likes the best.

Enrichment Activity C: Make 5 affirmation cards for a mama client.

The cards can be Scripture focused, Christian focused, mama preference focused, consider what you like or consider a pregnant mama friend to participate. If you choose a pregnant mama friend to participate, make sure you listen to her needs for the 5 cards you produce.

Please take a picture of the cards you make and submit to us via email if taking this for our doula course. Otherwise just make it for fun and use! Email to instructor.

<u>More on Christian or Catholic Spirituality:</u>

I am adding this in to help mothers who are Christian or Catholic have a better spirituality of birth experience.

A Catholic mother may enjoy praying the Rosary together during labor. I have done this before, and many clients said it has been the "highlight" of their labor of offering their sufferings and praying the Hail Mary's together.

If working with a Christian mother, she may enjoy praying the Our Father with you together. Or reading Biblical passages from the Bible during labor.

If working with a Christian or Catholic mother, remember to include a 'spiritual plan' for her labor!

<u>Letting Go of Fears Assignment</u> (Please practice with a mother):

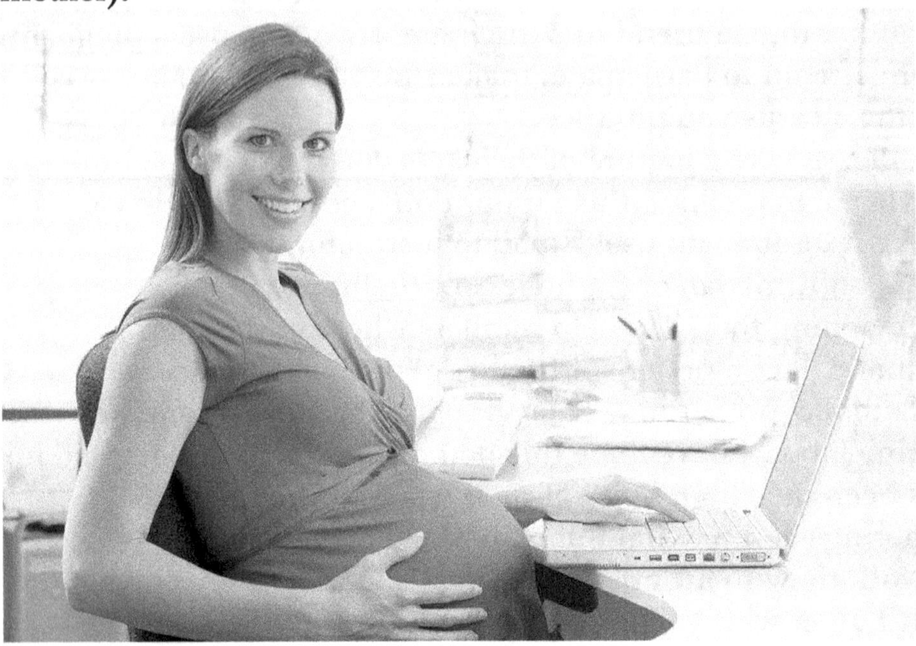

Letting go of Fears Exercise:

1. First of all have the mother sit down in a comfy chair and then write down a fear she has about childbirth. (If you are doing this and not pregnant – write down a different fear!)

2. Tell her to let go of the fear that is bothering her – have her repeat "I let go of this fear and give it to God."
3. Now take that piece of paper and either a) burn it b) throw it away if the burning thing is not something that would work for you. You can tear it up into little pieces if that helps before tossing it in the trash!

4. Now, have the mother sit and relax and have her do a breathing exercise (see later on in book for some techniques).
5. Ask the mother to turn her fears into hope – have her write down something like a positive thought, positive affirmation, etc.
6. Ask her how she feels after this – you may want to wait a week for her to practice this a few times before she responds.
7. If she still has fears, that also can be normal process of being pregnant. Fears may not go away in a day. Ask her to recite her affirmation or pray when she feels fearful.

(Do this exercise and turn in for credit to instructor).

Do this exercise with a mother if you can find one that is pregnant and turn it in for grade.

See our main classroom for quizzes as I am editing most of them for this edition of the book. Thank you.

Chapter 4: Pain, Childbirth, and the Bible

In our original version of this book, we did not really cover "pain" per se as a separate chapter. However, we wanted to add this in for this round of revision!

So, the most famous person that started research on Pain and Labor was Dick-Read. He came up with the idea of the Fear-tension-pain cycle. That women who have fears even if it is just fear of pain – will tense up and then have pain and then continue to do this cycle. In order to break the cycle, the woman needs to address the fears that she has. Sometimes these fears are also unknown.

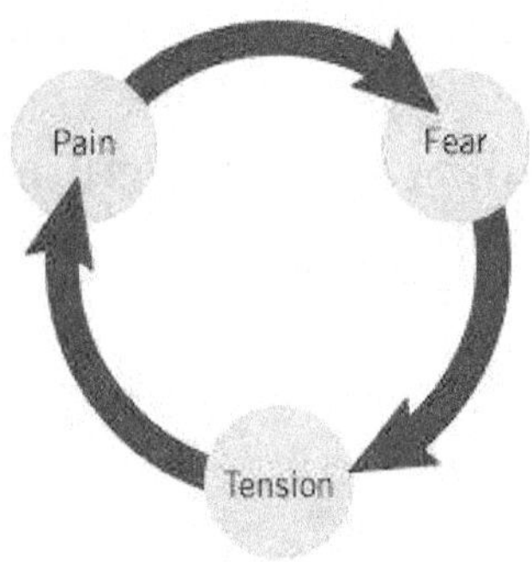

In an article titled "The Pain of Labor" by Andrea Robertson, she covers more about the role of Oxytocin during labor. Below from this article:

 She states: "Oxytocin is the hormone central to all aspects of reproductive behavior. In each area of reproduction (sexual intercourse, labor and birth, lactation) it works the same way and is affected by the same inhibiting factors."

 According to this article things such as nipple stimulation, cervix pressure, etc. will help oxytocin release. Things that inhibit oxytocin release include fear and anxiety, anesthetic injections, episiotomy, separation of mother and baby after birth, etc.

 Endorphins are natural pain killers especially during labor. The mother is hard at work and their numbers rise to help during times of stress. They help create a sense of well-being for the mother esp. after birth. They help support the mother and baby bonding after birth. Part of the reason a mother feels great after birth is due to endorphins and oxytocin.

□ Natural oxytocin is better for mom then having the non-natural Pitocin.

One note; Some mothers can cope with pain better than others. If you are also a childbirth educator; sometimes during a class, the educator will have the mother put ice on her arm and see how long she tolerates that, for instance. Anyway, if you have a mother who is unsure how well she tolerates pain or not – try the ice method or have her write down instances when she was in pain and how she responded! However, do remember that labor pain is a bit different – the body needs to have the mentality that this "pain" will end soon. Sometimes there are mothers who feel little or no pain. The idea of our method is to ease pain to the minimum as much as possible or to distract the mother into a calming relaxing birth time; so that when it is over, she won't even notice!

Another technique to try out is talking with the mother about fears and labor in the way below:

Talk to the Woman in Pain during labor by asking:

□ Is the woman talking through contractions?

□ Is she breathing well?

Does she need minimal coaching? Intense coaching?

□ Is she requesting pain relief?

□ Does the woman feel that there is adequate pain relief or that her pain is controlled?

Is reassurance and encouragement being given?

□ Another thing is you can ask the mother:

□ What's going on in the mother's mind? (What do you feel or see in your mind right now?)

What do you think will help?
What's wrong?
Is there something you are afraid of?
(Borrowed from Polly Perez)

If she confesses a fear – then attempt to have her "let, go of the fear" as in the above exercise "letting go of fears." However, doing this before labor may help better than during labor.

Biblical aspects of Pain!

Ephesians 6:6-14

[6] Let no man deceive you with vain words. For because of these things cometh the anger of God upon the children of unbelief. [7] Be ye not therefore partakers with them. [8] For you were heretofore darkness, but now light in the Lord. Walk then as children of the light. [9] For the fruit of the light is in all goodness, and justice, and truth; [10] Proving what is well pleasing to God: [11] And have no fellowship with the unfruitful works of darkness, but rather reprove them. [12] For the things that are done by them in secret, it is a shame even to speak of. [13] But all things that are reproved, are made manifest by the light; for all that is made manifest is light. [14] Wherefore he saith: Rise thou that steepest and arise from the dead: and Christ shall enlighten thee.

I know that passage does not sound much about pain – but think about it if we are children of God and children of light – then God is going to get us through pain of all kinds no matter how we feel.

Here is a longer website information on suffering: https://www.catholicnewsagency.com/resource/55695/st-paul-explains-the-meaning-of-suffering
In part of the above suffering article St. Paul says: "Indeed I count everything as loss because of the surpassing worth of knowing Christ Jesus my Lord. For his sake I have suffered the loss of all things, and count them as refuse, in order that I may gain Christ

and be found in him, not having a righteousness of my own, based on law, but that which is through faith in Christ, the righteousness from God depends on faith; that I may know him and the power of his resurrection, and may share his suffering, becoming like him in his death, that if possible I may attain the resurrection from the dead" (Philippians 3:8-11) (Source above).

So, now we know that the pain in childbirth is a bit different. The pain will go away eventually. The body knows there is a meaning for this pain.

<u>Here is some information about the types of pain of childbirth:</u>

The first type of pain is associated with muscle contractions as the cervix is opening or dilating. During this part of childbirth, the rows of muscles in your uterus contract (shorten), pulling open the cervix. Most women describe this feeling as an extremely strong menstrual cramp-like feeling. It may be felt in the lower part of the uterus, the low back, or both.

The second type of sensation is a feeling of intense pressure as the baby gets lower and pushes on the muscles in the pelvis and on the bladder and rectum. The third type of pain, which occurs as the baby is being born, is a feeling of burning or stretching as the vagina and skin stretch to let the baby through.

https://www.takingcharge.csh.umn.edu/explore-healing-practices/holistic-pregnancy-childbirth/what-about-pain

<u>Explore More</u>: Research Biblical passages about pain. Find 3 passages you like the best and submit to instructor.

1.

2.

3.

Our method to help with pain:
C.A.L.M. Method

C = Christ and Comfort: We aim at offering our sufferings through the merits of Jesus on the Cross – and Comfort – by working on any comfort technique that will help the mother during the contractions or pain sensations. Try heat/cold/ice/rebozo/positioning things already mentioned and breathing (next chapter).
A = Allow. This means allow the pain – embrace the pain. Sometimes we fear things and we are not embracing the moment – it is hard – not easy to do – embrace the pain/fear/ and then let go of the pain/fear. Allow God to enter into that moment.
L = Love and Learn. Love is something that may be hard to do during "labor of a baby." However, say to your baby, "I love you, come on down." You may be surprised what will happen! Learn – learn the responses your body makes to love. Get the husband/birth partner to embrace the mother during this "Love" exchange.
M=Mother or Meditation: The mother is the center of the labor time. Meditation is meaningful to the moment. See if the mother can concentrate on an affirmation or meditation of the Rosary for instance (if working with a Christian or Catholic mother). Or she may want to focus on breathing techniques, etc. Encourage the mother to release any fears also during this time of laboring using this "CALM" method.

Also, think of the fuller *Comfort in Birth Method* acronym during pain time. What comfort measures can you do to help? *ice *heat *affirmations *birth positions *birth ball time *breathing * rebozo skills *relaxation techniques *Miles circuit *get the nurse to help *drinking/hydration – see rest of this manual for more on our method.

<u>What's the Miles Circuit?</u>
The miles circuit was invented by a doula to help mothers and movement get the baby into a better position. You can read more here: http://www.milescircuit.com/the-circuit.html

1st. Step to Miles circuit is "Open-Knees chest". This is also helpful using a rebozo for this technique. The mother lies on her belly in this exercise and then lifts up her bottom and rests on her knees. I think a picture shows this technique the best:

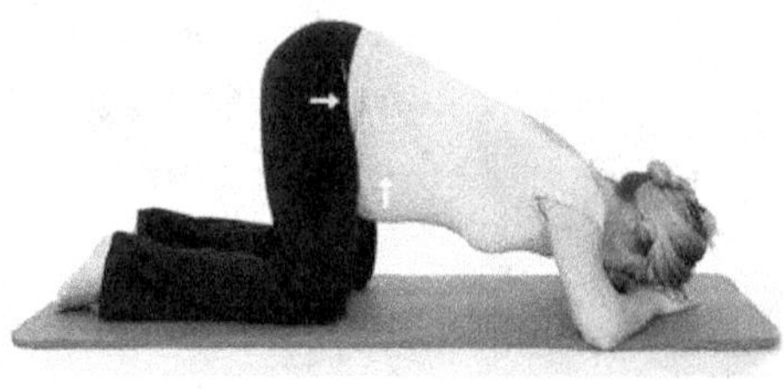

One can also use a *rebozo* (learn about rebozo Mexican shawl later in our book) to help hold up the mother's "buttocks" area and pull to help keep her stable. Not recommended if mother suffers from reflux. *Also, this position is good for a mother who might have cord prolapse.*

2nd Step of Miles circuit: Exaggerated side-lying position.

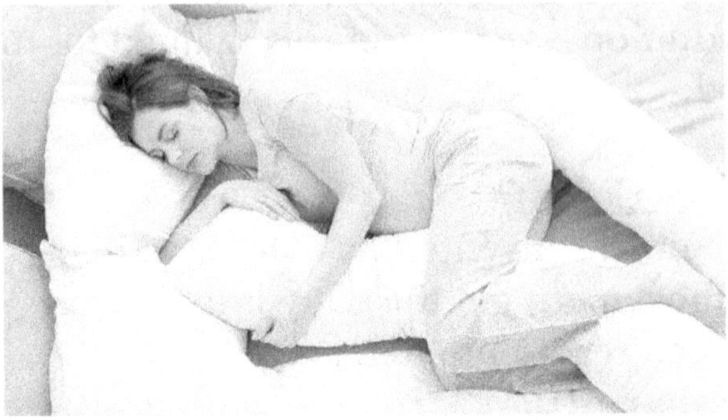

The mother may want some pillows for this one. She should attempt a side-lying position on a bed. She could also do this on a couch. Remember to switch sides if she goes through the miles circuit more than one time (which is recommended).

3rd Step of Miles circuit: Get moving! The author of Miles suggests doing a lunge, walking, going up stairs – however, in kind of a sidesway position – get someone to go up stairs behind mother.

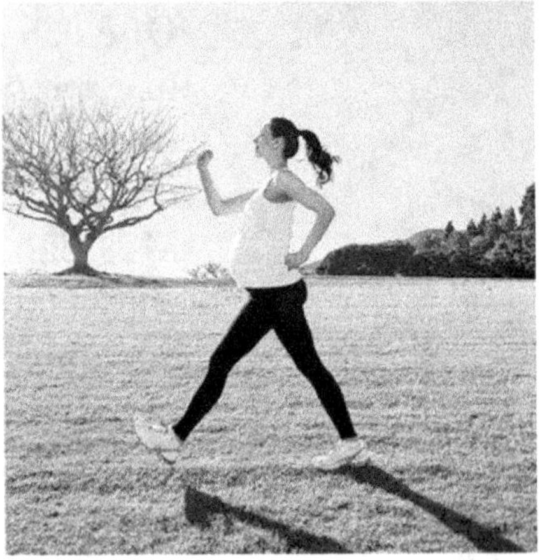

So, if you are working with a client, you may want to try the above as a practice run and skip the inversion if mother gets reflux.

Discuss the Miles circuit and send into instructor one thing you learned from this information.

I also found another website recently about Maternal optimal positioning – very similar sounding to miles – but maybe has more movements to consider. This is the website that explains more about this idea: https://www.optimalmaternalpositioning.com/whatisomp

We usually talk about baby positioning, but it also goes hand in hand with positioning *the mother* to certain ways to help her get the baby to come out better and faster. Here's another link about the optimal maternal positioning: https://www.optimalmaternalpositioning.com/omp-pelvic-mobility-protocols

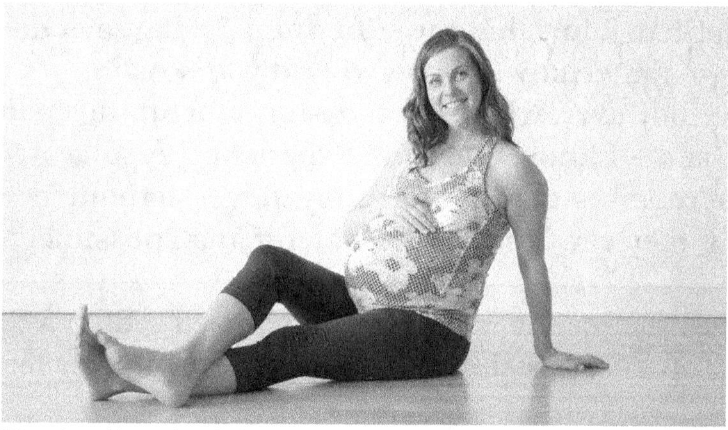

Basically, the idea is to put the mother in a good position for birthing her baby. It could be a good standing position or sitting or lying – whichever works for the moment. Also, preparation before she goes into labor is important with the techniques mentioned. Since some of this is beyond what we can print in our book right now, we hope you will explore the websites as well.

We hope this chapter was informative enough to help mothers in pain; some mothers may need extra help in the form of medication, and we need to reassure mothers that it is completely fine to get that epidural or pain medications for their birth. They should not feel like a failure just because they had an epidural, or the birth went south, and the mother had to get a c-section. We want to encourage mothers and validate their birth.

So, wrapping this up, Childbirth and pain is a normal process of labor, letting go of fears can help; also, get out the Bible and read! Next try out the Miles Circuit during labor esp. if things are not working so well. We hope this chapter on pain will help mothers know that the suffering is going to end – we cannot guarantee any method will rid you of pain completely – however, when you focus on other things pain seems to lessen – I know that from experience! Also, water can help – remember our "B" for Buoyancy – so mothers should ask if they can labor in the water if at all possible!

Assignment: Practice the Miles Circuit yourself – do it a few times. (Skip open knees chest if you have heartburn issues).

Case Study: Wendy is a mother who wants to practice a Christian way of keeping calm for pain. What can you suggest helping her? (Think of C.A.L.M. from this chapter – write out some tips or suggestions). Submit to instructor.

CHAPTER 5: What is a Nutritional doula? Plus Extra Bonus on ABC's of Birth Partner and Exercise

The goal of a nutritional doula is to help mothers eat "wholistically" and know what "real foods" vs. "junk food" are and more.

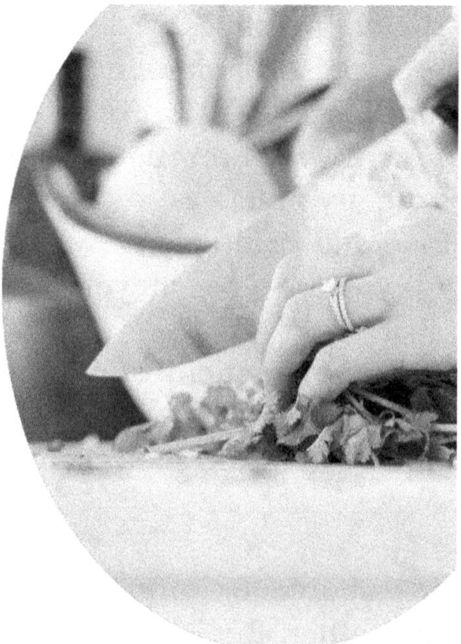

Nutritional Needs: A pregnant mother does not need to add in more calories the first trimester as long as she is getting in enough calories already based on a 2,100-calorie diet. When she is in second and third trimesters, she should be obtaining and increasing calories to 2,400 to 2,500 calorie diet.

Note: This eating goes by weight – so 1.2g of protein or more per kg of body weight. If she's not as active she might be able to get away with less – but this is a good average to consider. Yes, you will need to convert mama's weight into kilograms and then figure that out. Need help? Go to www.fabulousbodyacademy.com there's a calculator up there.

"Prematurity, low birth weight, long hard labor, premature rupture of membranes, placenta abruption, preeclampsia, fetal growth restriction, hypovolemia and hemorrhage can almost completely be prevented through proper attention to nutrition." ***By Midwifery Today article***[xxiii]

Nutrition is so important these days and many doctors do not discuss the importance of nutrition with their clients.

<u>What can a nutritional doula offer?</u>
A nutritional doula offers consultations to her mother client during pregnancy and/or postpartum time frame that help the mother find "whole/real food" dietary practices.
*She (nutritional doula) can offer in person or phone consultations and charge a fee for this.
*A nutritional doula may offer a pantry walk through and how to offer changes in the mother's dietary practices.
*A nutritional doula may offer food and menu plans (with permission from her doctor – or if you are a coach, you may not need this permission).
*A nutritional doula may even cook for her client! (For those bakers!)
*A nutritional doula helps with the postpartum food planning too!

You as a doula might be the only resource for information about nutrition for your pregnant mother. Remember *doctor's offices usually only see a mother for 15 minutes or so at a time. They are not going to address nutritional needs unless something is "wrong" already. *Midwives may go over nutrition more.
Preventive measures for this would be to know about nutrition first! So, don't be surprised if a mother asks you about her diet, etc. However, we do recommend that you obtain the nutritional doula full certification in order to be a nutritional specialist!

<u>What does a nutritional doula do?</u>

So, let's say you are sitting down with a mama client and talking about nutrition. What can you say or offer?

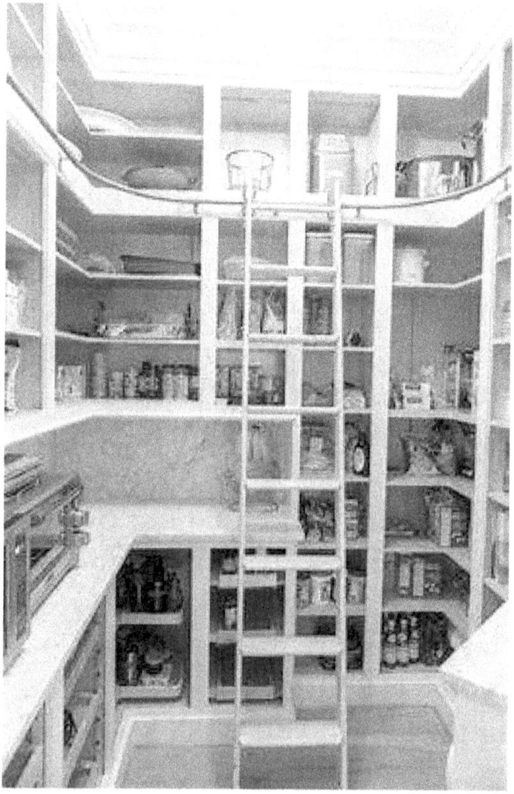

1. Unless you are a certified holistic nutritional coach (like your teacher) – you need to be careful what you say – make sure you are saying things like "suggested research shows that if a mother takes this or eats this food it will help with whatever." Make sure you can back up what you say with research.

2. You cannot suggest "diet" meal plans unless you are a coach or have a dietician background. You can suggest foods in general to eat – like the Brewer's diet, Whole Foods diet, etc. She will have to produce her own meal plan. (If you want a course that makes you a coach let us know). So, you can say this is a Whole Foods Meal plan that you could follow (for instance). Or get permission from her doctor to do more specific food plans.

3. You can sit down and go over her pantry and see what foods you would recommend adding to it. (Or throw it out – depending on her food needs). However, I would be cautious about throwing out things – let her suggest that she shouldn't eat as much sugar, etc. You might be surprised! So, you can do

a "pantry walk through" with her to see what foods are good and bad.

Macro vs. Micro…

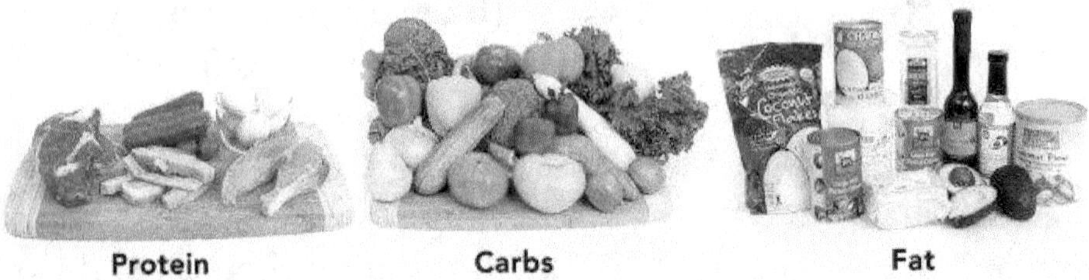

Macronutrients are the major foods that we need to eat in order to get by each day – things like proteins, fats, carbs, etc. So, this is your fish, chicken, beef, potatoes, vegetables, etc.

Micronutrients are the minerals and things like that our body needs everyday as well. This would be like calcium in milk for instance.

In our fuller nutritional class, we go over some pillars of nutrition and eat a rainbow of foods, etc.

So, if a mother wants something to eat and you don't know what to recommend, we suggest she eat a rainbow of foods.

<u>Help prevent moms becoming anemic…</u>

One thing a doula can support is after the end of the first trimester – the mother nutrients may be lower and she can make sure the mother is getting the extra protein and sodium in now.

Protein – building blocks of the baby!

Salt – Sodium

Iron – to avoid Anemia – An important milestone in the mother's pregnancy is week 28 is when the mother's blood volume doubles and she needs to make sure her hemoglobin (iron) levels are good and continue to be so the rest of the pregnancy.

Calcium – Important to eat away from iron products – so eat your meat without the cheese or milk – eat like a Jew during pregnancy – they do not eat their meat with milk or dairy product.

According to the author of *Birth Conspiracy*, "the best nutrition for mother is whole foods diet". We agree. Supplements are good to take; but having a whole foods diet is important to mother and baby.

Also, the author discusses in this chapter "What is nourishment?" There is a diet called the "Brewer's Diet" that is a good one for mothers to follow. Look up more information by doing your own research.

*Discuss three things you learned from this section so far and turn into teacher.

1.
2.
3.

__What is a Whole Foods[xxiv] diet?__

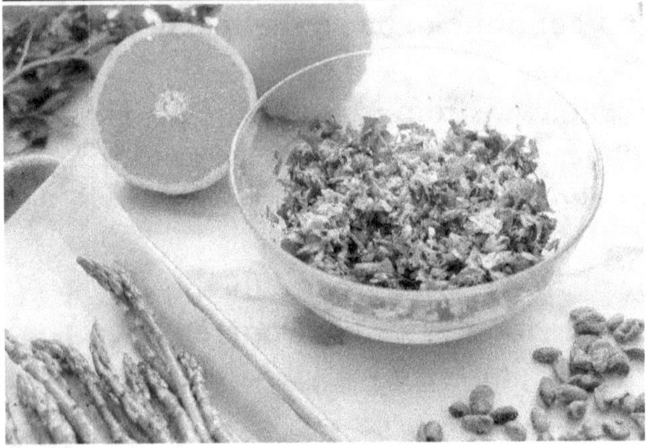

Usually this means:
"Eating organically or no-GMO" as much as possible.
Eating whole grains. Brown Rice vs. White Rice for instance.
Eating beef, chicken, turkey, fish – from healthy sources if possible.
Also, drinking keifer, kombucha, etc.
Eating healthy vegetables—organic or from a Farmer's market first.
Drinking healthy water – Reverse Osmosis, Distilled (add in minerals), spring water, etc.
Drinking other things like natural orange juice, etc.

__Eating during laboring time:__

Most hospitals have a no-eat policy, though this is changing in some areas. When you do your hospital visit (part of your certification requirement)—ask your local hospital if they allow eating during labor.

Nourishment is important for mothers during labor. If she cannot have regular foods, encourage her to suck on a honey stick; take in juices; or bring her own food if that is allowed.

A mother may get tired or exhausted just because she has not eaten in 12-24 hours depending on length of labor.
Also, encourage clients to eat before going to hospital if possible.
For some reason, I personally just can't eat much during labor and some moms maybe like that too!

What to do if a hospital says "no" to eating during labor?
If your hospital has a no eat during labor policy – suggestions:
Get all the ice chips you can at the hospital.
Stay at home longer and eat at home before heading to the hospital. This is probably the best advice – you can eat while at your home and then make sure you are well hydrated at the hospital when you get there.
Sneak food in and eat it anyway!!
Get a protein drink made up and labor aide tea – drink this during labor!
Labor aide drink recipe:
https://www.baby-chick.com/labor-aide-recipe/
https://mommypotamus.com/how-to-make-a-labor-aid-electrolyte-drink/
https://documentingsimpleliving.com/labor-aid-recipe/
Practice making one for fun or make one for our case study in this section.

Case Study Charlotte
Charlotte is a new mother and wants a labor aide drink recipe. Can you find her one? Also, make the labor aide drink recipe if you have time (for extra credit). Submit to instructor.
Discussion over this section of the chapter:
For Discussion: What is a nutritional doula?
What does a nutritional doula do?

What does a proper diet include for pregnancy?
For lactation?
What can you offer mothers as a nutritional doula?
What about eating during labor?
Please submit it to the instructor!

More on Nutrition – What to eat or not eat?

First of all mothers are told to "NOT" eat a lot of foods. And if you or your client has additional health issues it may make it harder for them to know what to eat or not eat during pregnancy. A mother with gestational diabetes may need to limit carbs. A mother with gluten intolerance will also not be eating wheat or gluten products. A more Paleo diet approach may work more for these mothers. We are not going to cover what not to eat "so to speak" – instead we want to cover more on what to eat to help mothers out.
Second, another thing to consider is who's your target market (for doulas)? Are you working with a mother who can afford organic foods and such or not? Some mothers may not have the finances to eat properly in some instances. If your client is lower income, then you will need to help her make "healthy" choices at her local supermarket vs. natural grocery store. Encourage all mothers to read labels and understand what GMO means (genetically modified organism in foods). Encourage mothers to choose something else when possible. Encourage low-income mothers to shop the sales and know how to find food deals or clip coupons too!
Thirdly, even a low-income mother may be able to shop at a local farmer's market. A local farmers market usually happens in most towns throughout the summer. Encourage your client to look for and buy from local farmers. Sometimes a low-

income mother can get vouchers for free local farmer market food depending on the city she lives in. Encourage mothers to look into this idea.

Asian Traditions of Eating for Pregnancy:

Seven Guidelines:

1. Eat Real Food!
   Like we mentioned above go to the local farmer's market and obtain healthier grown foods for you and your family as a pregnant mother. Fresh foods are so much better for a mother than non-fresh. Also, if you can drink dairy milk then you might be able to find raw milk or raw goat's milk if you prefer goat milk. Almonds, coconut, and dates are also known as "sattvic" foods as they help nourish the body better esp. during pregnancy. Remember to read labels and see what ingredients are in them if you do pick up a boxed food item. Is this something you want to put in your body? Do you understand what GMO's are? Do you understand what monosodium glutamate does?
2. Eat Protein with Every Meal or Snack? Why?

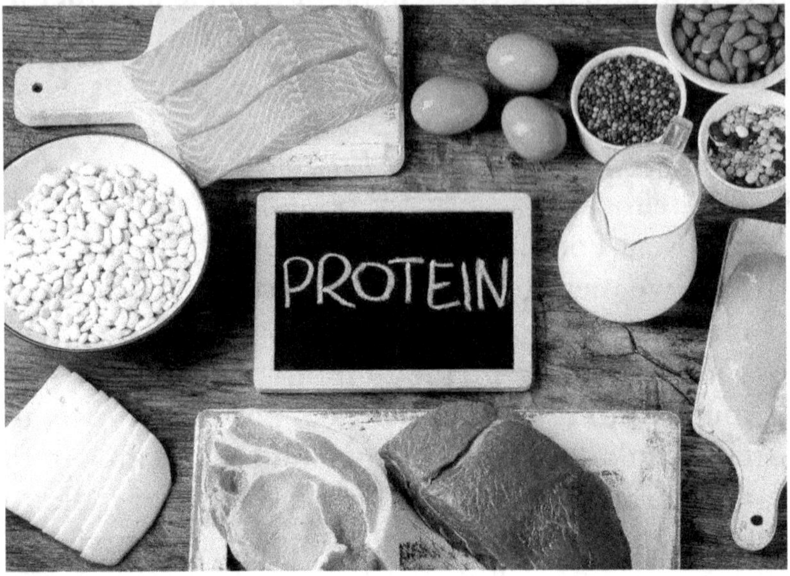

Because most mothers do not get enough protein in their diet as pregnant mothers. "Protein helps regulate blood pressure during pregnancy, thanks to amino acid glycine."(Nine Golden Months). "Glycine also protects against oxidative stress that is a hallmark of preeclampsia."[xxv]

What are protein sources? First of all beef, chicken, turkey, lamb, venison, bison, etc. Second, fish and shrimp and any sea creatures! Third, Milk, dairy, eggs. Fourth, alternatives for vegans would be beans and rice (complete protein), quinoa (has protein in it), tofu, tempeh, etc. Fifth, Nuts also have some protein in them. Encourage mothers to eat nut butters if they don't have an allergy to it! Bone broth is also a good source of nutrients for mothers to eat.

3. Fill Your plate with abundance of vegetables (and fruits):

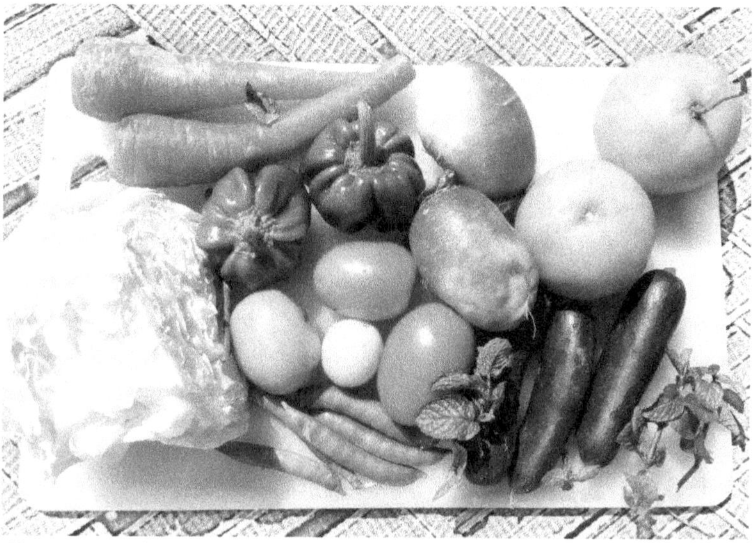

Get creative in making vegetables a part of your everyday life as a pregnant mother. Doulas should encourage mothers to eat a "rainbow" of foods. Prebiotic type foods include asparagus, artichoke, jicama, leeks, onions, palm hearts, leeks, and apples. Prebiotics mean the food can help restore your gut function better. This is also important for pregnancy. If you have better gut function, then less problems with depression. Mothers should also eat food like broccoli, brussel sprouts, green beans, yellow squash, butternut squash, oranges, grapes, lemons, tomatoes (if not allergic), etc. Basically eat a rainbow! Another thing, a mother can eat fermented foods to help with the gut function we mentioned above. So, she can eat sauerkraut, yogurt (try to get no sugar added type), pickles, and relishes. Kombucha should be done in moderation since it does have some caffeine in it – might be a good alternative to coffee!

4. Embrace the Good Fats! What's a good fat?

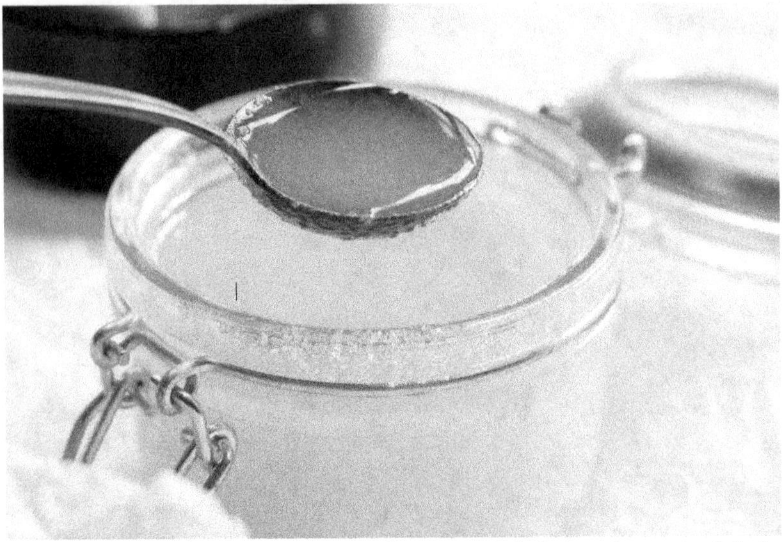

Believe it or not – butter is a good fat, ghee (which is clarified butter if you want something healthier), avocado oil, coconut oil, good quality lard or tallow (you can also home make this one), virgin olive oil. Any other "oil" is going to be lesser quality and not as good for you. Palm oil is one of the worst fats you can eat. Also, vegetable oils are not good for you, and they usually have corn oil in them which is GMO. So, avoiding vegetable oils would be a good thing. If you are a pregnant mother reading this and thinking, "Oh, no, all I have is vegetable oil" then go out and shop for some of these other oils right now!

5. Reduce your sugar intake significantly: Why? It will help prevent gestational diabetes from beginning with and your body will benefit from less sugar. You can try alternatives – but be careful – do not eat sweeteners that are artificially made. Stevia, monk fruit, agave, honey, etc. are examples of alternatives.

6. Stay Hydrated. A good aim for pregnant mothers is 8-10 glasses (8 ounces each) a day. You are building a baby and you have amniotic fluid to keep up and it helps your baby grow if you are taking in enough fluids. You can also stay hydrated with soups, stews, fresh vegetables, and fruits too. Doula tip: Mother "roasting" can begin in pregnancy – mothers need to keep warm even during pregnancy. If mothers eat warming soups and stews then this will help their spleen stay happy and keep their bodies in balance up to postpartum. By postpartum the mother will be used to eating soups and stews which are great for recovery!
7. *Remember to eat as "kindly as you can".* Do your best as a mother to take all of these ideas and run with them. This is your time to enjoy food, not think of it as a chore. Experiment with various recipes. In fact we recommend Heng Ou's new book "Nine Golden Months" as a book to read about nutrition and various recipes are in the back of that book for cooking! Remember to also try to avoid pesticides in foods. Go to this website: ewg.org to get a list of foods that are commonly grown with pesticides in them. At least rinse your fruits and veggies before eating!

*****There will be a quiz over this chapter! See end of chapter.***

Enrichment Assignment – Food diary!

Challenge: Ask 3 people about their food intake for 3 days. Ideas try to vary up this list of people. For instance: ask a teenager, ask a pregnant mother, ask a lactating mother. Have them fill out the form (see appendix of Comfort in Birth Method book) for diary for nutrition. After reviewing the chart of their eating for 3 days. What do you think is missing in their diets? Remember protein, carbs, vegetables/fruits are important. Think of it as a plate. The protein and vegetables/fruits should be more than carbs for instance. Sweets should be minimal. Also, dairy products can be included too. Consider at least one item that they could do to help their diet. Suggest it to the participants.

Food diary should be at least 5 days.
It should list Breakfast Foods, Lunch Foods, and supper foods. It also should list drinks the participant drank those days (appx. How many cups as well.)
You may look it over and offer one "suggested" change to participant if so desired.
Send to instructor the food diary and any suggested changes. Thank you.

Extra Bonus for this Chapter: ABC's of Being a Good Birth Partner:

A: Allow yourself to be the best partner you can be!
A doula is a type of birth partner – but there are other birth partners too:
If a dad is the only one supporting the mother, he should be encouraged to be the "best birth partner" as much as possible as well.
Friends and relatives can also be "birth partners" when a mother is in labor and helps a mom give birth.
There are a variety of birth partners. Doulas are "trained" birth partners, but we should encourage family members to participate in birth as well.
**Discussion: "What kind of birth partner are you?" What qualities make you a good doula?

B: Being hired by the mother:
A mother will usually put down about 50 percent of the doula fee when hiring the doula. The rest of the balance is due

before birth. Therefore, it is important for mothers to learn and hire a doula earlier on – as many doulas offer payment plans. Some also offer military discounts or may take a lower down payment.

After being hired, the doula will usually arrange for the first meeting – and make sure her client understands the doula contract. The doula may meet at the mother's home or if the doula has an office – the mom may meet there as well.

At the first meeting the mother will fill out a "Mother Enrichment" Form or a "Form" about the mother's health and any previous births or miscarriages. We have a sample intake form in the back of this book.

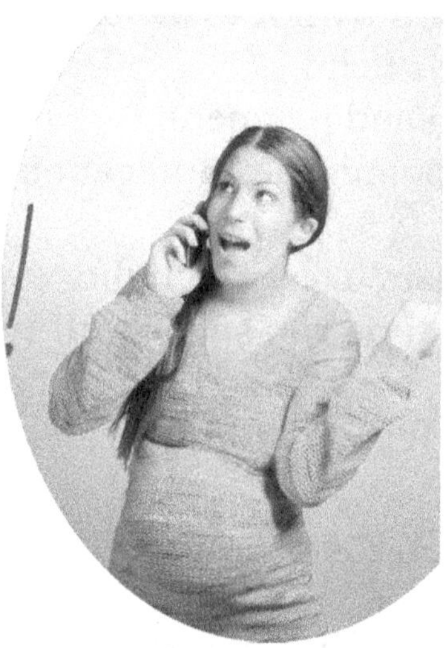

__Being hired includes meeting the mother:__ 1st Contact: The first contact with a prospective client is often a very important one. She will be trying to find out what kind of person you are, perhaps what a doula is, and she will have questions and concerns.

Phone or Email: Set up a time to properly meetup.

A zoom call can also be made if so desired or regular phone call.

After the meeting, follow-up but be patient to let the person make a decision. However, it is appropriate to remind them that your schedule fills up fast and give them a deadline for a decision. (This works even if you are new, and your schedule is wide open!)

If the person is not responding, it might be time to move on; however, sending an email a week or two out after your first contact is appropriate. If they respond to say they made a decision to go with someone else, don't take it too hard. However, you might also surprise the client by saying you just filled their spot! (If that is the case – I hope they regret not acting faster!)

What if you cannot find clients? Check out my book "Doing Business the Doula Way."

You are hired now what:

*Make sure she knows how to reach you 24/7, so when she goes into labor, she's got you on speed dial!

*Keep open communication with your mom. Ask how she's doing? Ask how you can help her?

*Keep prenatal appointments with her and try not to cancel.

*Help her with her birth plan if she needs help!

*Let her know your contract information and payment information up front. That way there is no miscommunication or hurt feelings later.

*We recommend a non-refundable deposit. That way if the client backs out, you are covered for the time you spent with them. The only time to offer a refund on this is if a client had a miscarriage—then it would be nice to offer a full refund.

C is for Childbirth Education and Birth Wishes:

The doula usually offers 2 prenatals.

The first one may cover "Birth wishes" or "Birth plans" which we will cover more in another module. The second meeting will most likely cover comfort measures for labor and be a small educational time for the mother.

However, remember you are NOT a childbirth educator. If the mother is obviously un-educated in the birth processes – we suggest that you obtain Childbirth Educator status and then

offer this as a bonus to mothers – even one-on-one classes for her.
We recommend Magnificat Childbirth Educator course – ask us for info.
http://www.catholicdoula.com/childbirtheducation.html

C for Confidentiality
Remember to keep your client's information Confidential – look up the new HIPPA requirements if needed.
Using the right language at birth and when meeting with the parents.
Using the word "vagina" may be vulgar to a mother. Ask her if she's OK with "yoni" or some other term.
"Letting your bottom open – may sound better if you say: let your body flower open".
She may not want the doctor being the one "delivering the baby" when she's doing all the work… "Let your body flow down and receive your baby" will sound a lot better!!

ABC- Also be flexible for mother's schedules:
*Try to be flexible with the mom's needs.
*Give her your back-up doula info—if you have one.
*Take care of your mom! Do your part to show up on time; be courteous on the phone. And by the way if someone judges you by your phone messages left – my advice—don't leave a detailed message with anyone. Just leave your name/phone number to get back with you. This way you can meet in person. I find phone personality can differ than in person for sure!
Discussion: Discuss this section about being prepared as a doula for helping moms, etc.

V for Visiting the hospital or Birth Center:

The birth partner (usually the father and doula can also do this) should visit the mother's care giver/doctor or midwife and establish the final details of the birth plan.

The birth partner visits the hospital or birth center.

The mother should pre-register at the hospital or birth center to make sure.

Arrange for the doula to be with the mother at the hospital or birth center.

The Birth Partner book also covered this. So, you may want to go back and look at Chapter 1-2 again.

**Requirement: Learn about the current "doula" policies in your hospital. Do they require doulas to have a certificate? Do they require you to wear mask? What else may they require? Also, check out the "guests" policies. Are they less restrictive? Could you get away with being a "guest" as a doula for a birth? What works best for your business model?

Submit to instructor if you are taking this class for credit.

Another thing to consider is working with midwives and birth centers.

Find a midwife in your area who would work with a doula. What are her requirements for going to a birth center birth?

Also, you may want to have a backup doula just in case you need one. A backup doula helps you when you need to go home during labor to rest especially if it is an extremely long labor – sometimes babies do not come fast, so having a backup doula can help you get a break if needed during laboring time too.

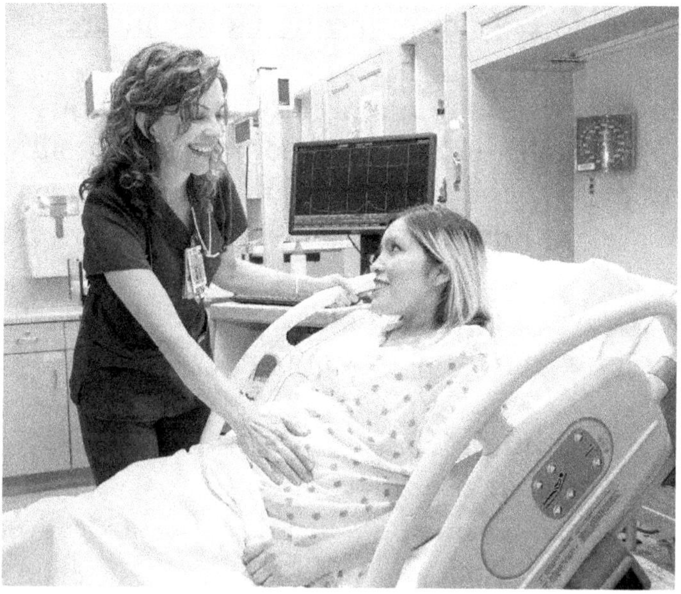

ABC-B for Doula Bag – what's in your doula bag assignment:
**What's in YOUR Doula Bag?
Time to start your doula bag collection.
Put together a doula bag of tricks so to speak.
What items would you put in your bag?
Send in a picture of your bag **AND** items inside. Send a list of items too. If you cannot get a bag, at least try to put together some items you would put in a bag.
Think of comfort measure kinds of items a mother may want – if you need to read ahead to think about that and come back to this assignment that is great.
Here are some ideas: massage tool, rice sock (to get cold or heat up), birth ball, rebozo, a small fan, affirmation cards, positioning cards (for reminder – can find at Plum Tree Baby), etc. Submit your doula bag picture or list of items to instructor or see appendix for more tips on this assignment.

CHAPTER 6: Listening & Communication and Cultures

We are expanding this section a little more from the previous edition in order to make our program more compatible for all doulas to have a better experience in your education. Mothers may read through as well to understand this better too.

In this section we will cover 3 types of listening sections:

1. Active listening and some tips on how to accomplish this.
2. Inter-professional communication.
3. Cross-cultural communication.
4. Our Cultural Advocacy Project
5. Quiz over chapter for doulas in training.

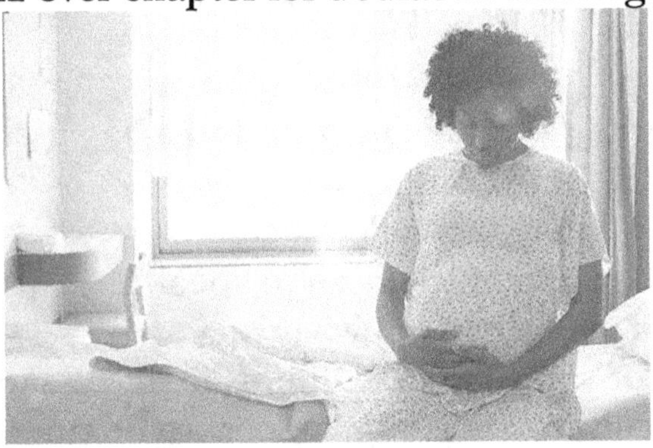

Communicating with laboring women is important – here's a short article that may help you learn more: Read this article: https://nursekey.com/communicating-with-laboring-women/ The main point of this article is that a lot of doctors do things and they only say "I am going to check you"; but do not explain why! So, if you are a doula in the room during a "check you moment," you can tell the doctor something like: "Can you explain to my client or the mother why you are checking her and what you are going to be doing right this minute?" This way the mother has more knowledge about what is happening, and you are "advocating" for her rights to know.

**Discuss one thing you learned from the laboring woman article.

<u>Active Listening:</u>

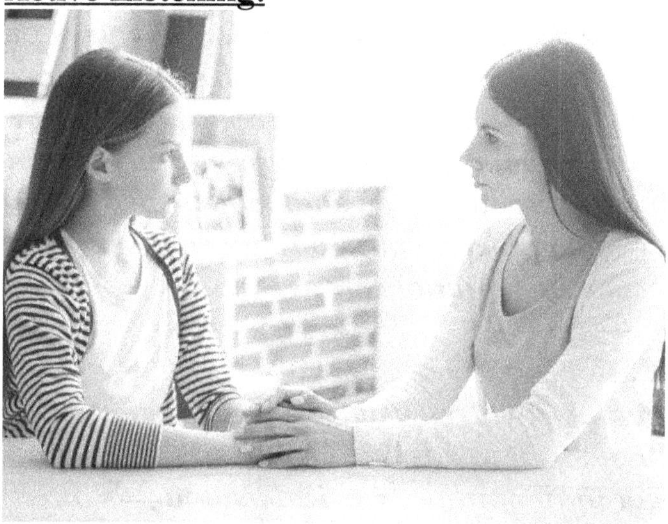

Active listening is important for doulas as we are going to be communicating with clients, nurses, doctors, midwives, and even other doulas in our business. We should take time to know how to actively communicate better by listening first.

Before we get into the various tips that we can offer, first we want to go over 4 types of listening that exist.

> Quoted article: *1. Deep Listening*
> *Deep listening occurs when you're committed to understanding the speaker's perspective. It involves paying attention to both verbal and nonverbal cues, such*

as the words being used, the speaker's body language, and their tone. This type of listening helps build trust and rapport, and it helps others feel comfortable in expressing their thoughts and opinions.

2. Full Listening
Full listening involves paying close and careful attention to what the speaker is conveying. It often involves the use of active listening techniques, such as paraphrasing what's been said to the person, you're speaking with to ensure you understand their messaging. Full listening is useful in the classroom, when someone is instructing you on how to complete a task, and when discussing work projects with superiors.

3. Critical Listening
Critical listening involves using systematic reasoning and careful thought to analyze a speaker's message and separate fact from opinion. Critical listening is often useful in situations when speakers may have a certain agenda or goal, such as watching political debates, or when a salesperson is pitching a product or service.

4. Therapeutic Listening
Therapeutic listening means allowing a friend, colleague, or family member to discuss their problems. It involves emphasizing and applying supportive nonverbal cues, such as nodding and maintaining eye contact, in addition to empathizing with their experiences. (End of quote)[xxvi]

Active Listening Tips:

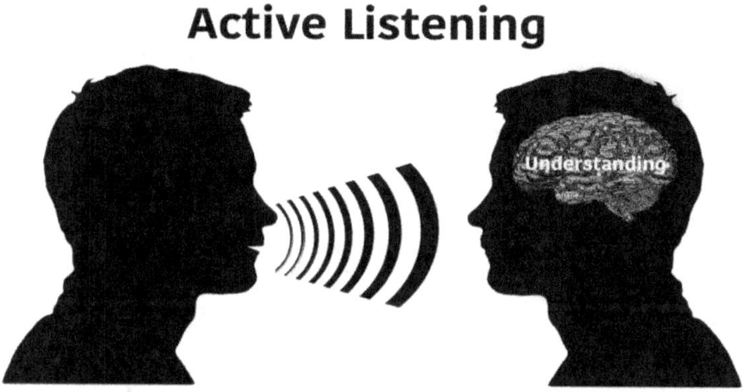

1. *Paraphrase*
   Once "a mother client" has finished expressing a thought, paraphrase what (she) said to make sure you understand and to show that you are paying attention. Things you can say are "What I hear you saying is...," "It sounds like...," or "If I understand you right...."[xxvii]
2. *Ask questions.*
   When appropriate, ask questions to encourage the (mother) to elaborate on their thoughts and feelings. Try to avoid jumping to conclusions about what is being said. Instead, ask questions such as, "When you say_____, do you mean_____?" to clarify their meaning.
3. *Use body language.*
   As the listener, show that you are engaged and interested by nodding, facing the other person, and maintaining an open and relaxed body posture. Try to avoid attending to distractions in your environment or checking your phone. In addition, be mindful of your facial expressions. Avoid expressions that might convey disapproval.

4. Show empathy. If the (mother) voices negative feelings, try to validate them rather than question them. Try to consider why they feel this way and put yourself in their shoes. You could say, "I can understand how that situation could cause frustration."

5. *Avoid judgement.*
   Your goal is to understand your (mother's) perspective. Try not to interrupt with your own opinions while the student is speaking. Getting emotionally involved, angry, or upset is something you don't want to do. You are a role model, and (mothers) are looking up to you (since you are a doula).
6. *Avoid giving advice too quickly.*
   Allow the (mother) to finish speaking before attempting to give advice. You want to make sure that you fully understand them first. Moving too quickly into advice-giving can be counterproductive.
7. *Evaluate*
   After you have fully interpreted what the (mother) has said, take a moment to evaluate the conversation.
8. *Know that just listening is sometimes enough.*
   Sometimes (mothers) just want someone to listen to them. As (doulas), we tend to want to "fix" our (mothers' problems) for them. But if our minds are busy coming up with solutions for them, we fail to truly listen.

Active listening takes thought, practice, and a desire to put your (mother's) feelings above your own. Using active listening skills can make a meaningful difference in a (mother's) life. (End of quoted article – we replaced the words "students" and "teachers" to be "mothers" and "doula" in this article for better relevancy).[xxviii]

Discussion: Please discuss 2 tips you learned from the above article(s). Does this help you understand active listening better?

*Active Listening Assignment:

Pretend this scenario below:

Lisa is a new mother and scared about giving birth in a hospital. She does not like this idea, but her insurance will not cover home birth. She wants some reassurance about giving birth naturally in a hospital. One of you pretends to be Lisa and the other person pretends to be the doula – act out some questions that maybe Lisa has – practice active listening to Lisa's questions and concerns. Wait before replying – practice the above techniques as you respond as a doula. Work on this scenario for a few minutes.

What to submit for assignment – if you can record yourself and a friend playing out scenario bonus points – otherwise submit a paragraph or two about how well you did. Were you able to capture most of the tips from above when active listening? Did you ever interrupt the mother, not do something right? Minus a point for each infraction! Submit your two paragraphs for grading. Make sure you cover the points mentioned in the tips above. Thank you.
Remember to email to comfortinbirth@gmail.com or catholicdoulanews@gmail.com

Interprofessional Communication: What does this mean?

First of all, this means being professional in communicating with a client. Leaving personal feelings of your day out of the conversation. Here's a good example: "How are you doing?" It might be better to say, "I am fine," to a client even if you are having a bad day – it would sound a lot better than "my neck and back hurt."

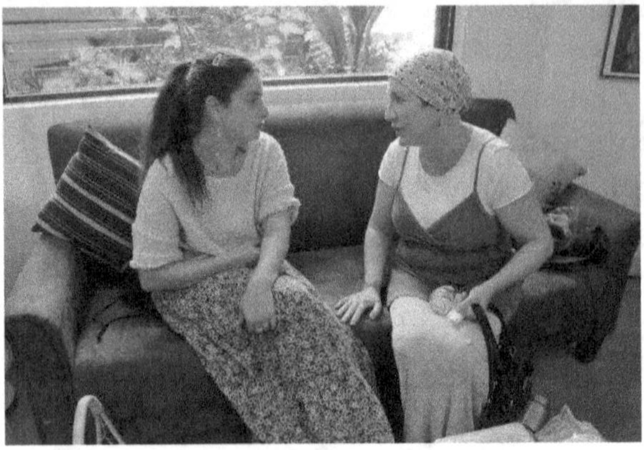

Second, we should also be professional doctors and nurses that cross our path. We want them to have a positive experience with you as a doula. If you are working at a particular hospital that has had "bad doulas", you need to change their mind about that and see how "bright" and "grateful" you are to be able to work alongside these staff. Be polite, say "Thank you." Ask what name they would like to be addressed as "Doctor…" or "Nurse…" Remember they are the ones in charge and always ask the nurse like, "Can we move this or that to help make my client more comfortable." Or "Can you help me get my client on a birth ball – she would like to use one right now." Etc.

Third, don't take charge of a situation that is not yours to decide. Always advocate for the mother, but not get in way of emergencies, etc. Let's say the staff wants to tie down and cut umbilical cord right away. You can say, "Did the mother consent to having the umbilical cord cut right away? Can we ask her if she wants to wait a few minutes? Is there a medical reason why the umbilical cord should be cut now?" Perhaps the staff will back off. If they have already clamped, it – maybe you can still buy her a minute – clamping does not mean blood stops pulsating – it will only stop once it is cut for instance. Anyway, no matter what the scenario is about – be professional and not get in the way. The nurse's reply may vary and if it is a true emergency, you are not going to want to get in the way!

Fourth, If there is a true emergency, wait for it to be settled and get out of the way. It is better to do that than the staff not wanting you to come back to a hospital.

Fifth, interprofessional communication means that you are professional while still able to communicate what the client needs or wants – plus, make sure the client can speak up for herself. If she's able to talk at that moment, let the staff know, "My client wants to tell you something once her contraction is over," for instance. It is better if the mother advocates for herself and you are there as kind of her guidepost.

Six – Here's an articles you can read more about interprofessional communication: https://www.indeed.com/career-advice/career-development/interprofessional-collaboration#:~:text=Collaborating%20as%20a%20team%20and,assess%20and%20diagnose%20the%20issue.

Second article: https://www.ncbi.nlm.nih.gov/pmc/articles/PMC6387781/#:~:text=Interprofessional%20(IP)%20communication%20describes%20the,either%20be%20intentional%20or%20unintentional.

Third article: https://pressbooks.library.torontomu.ca/communicationnursing/chapter/interprofessional-communication/#:~:text=Written%20communication%20in%20the%20interprofessional,%2C%20and%20more%20recently%2C%20texts.

**Discuss one thing you learned from one of the above communication articles and one thing you learned from our take on professional communication.

Cross-Cultural Communication

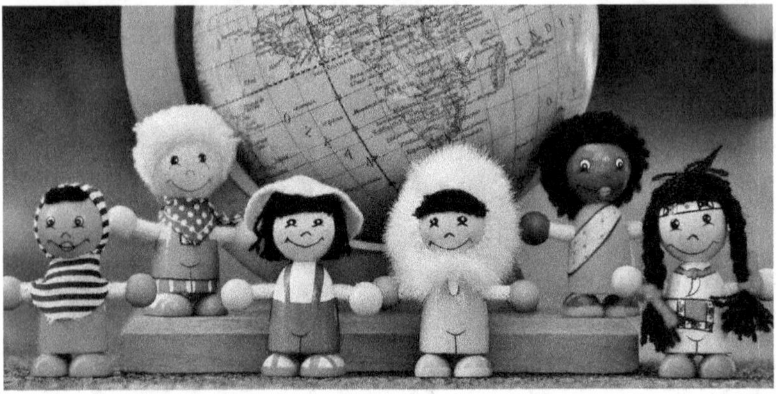

1. This may be one of the hardest ones to define or consider. Cross-cultural communication is communication across cultures, races, languages, or other barriers.
2. Various cultures even use hand gestures differently than we do. If you have a habit of talking and using your hands as well, then you may end up telling someone in another country "to eat mice for lunch" – or whatever weird thing that might come up. So, when speaking with someone from another culture, it is best not to use your hands when communicating – to avoid any unpleasant misinterpretation.
3. Perhaps you may need to have someone translate for you at a hospital or other place when working with a client. If your client's husband is deaf for instance, then you may need someone there to translate ASL to English for you. If you have a client that is only Spanish speaking, you may need a relative to convey what you are saying to them from your native tongue of English (or unless you speak another language). Remember to follow the rules

of active listening when working with cultural communication. This might be a key ingredient.

4. Repeat what the person said and then add your own thoughts at the end. This will help the person from another culture understand that you understood what they said, and you are confirming it, etc.
5. Be sensitive to your client's needs in communication. If the person knows how to Write and Read English better than speaking it – you also may want to try that out for communicating as a team effort.
6. In labor time, the mother may not be able to communicate as well, so maybe make up hand signals that mean various things – it will be a fun way to communicate and if you have figured all this out before the birth – then she will appreciate the time you spent learning this. You could learn some ASL even if so desired.
7. Whatever way you decide to communicate across cultures, remember to respect the way the client wants their birth done. Perhaps, they are supposed to be quiet throughout the birth – then help the mother and support her in that quiet strength of labor.
8. If you have had a miscommunication and don't understand, make sure you have a sign or indicator or just tell her you don't understand and maybe get help for the mother to get better communication.
9. If you are concerned about an upcoming birth with someone from another culture, remember to tell the hospital staff and see how they can help, for instance. Or if the mother is having a homebirth – then you can communicate this to the midwife, etc.

10. Learning about the culture you are working with is important too. If the mother is from a country, you are unfamiliar with their pregnancy and childbirth practices, then you may want to do some research and find out more about what they believe in.
11. Also, a mother may not practice her cultural or religious practices at all – make sure you ask her – if she has something specific for her religion or culture that she wants you to help with at birth. She may tell you that she does not want to do certain things, etc. Don't assume she's practicing her religion or culture until you ask – make it part of your intake form, so it won't offend anyone. You can put a little section on your intake form something like "Do you have any culture practices you wish to add to your birth or birth plan?" Or "Do you have any religious practices you wish to add to your birth plan?" This way it helps you know one way or the other way before the birth!

Discuss: Discuss 2 things you learned about helping cultures and communication.

<u>Cultural Birth Advocacy Project</u>

Being a "Comfort in Birth" Doula also means becoming an advocate for the mother. An advocate listens, understands, and knows what the mother desires for her upcoming birth. An advocate listens, understands and helps the mother know about the doctor or midwife's requests during labor. An advocate helps the mother be more informed at birth.

Cultural Advocacy:

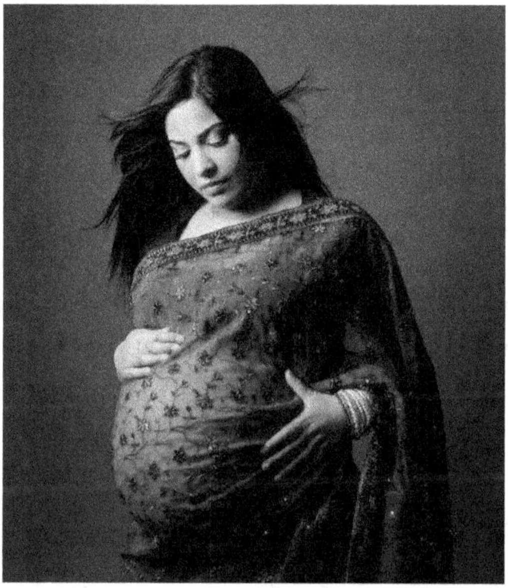

Part of our listening and advocacy means we need to understand the cultures of birth. Mothers from various cultures have various beliefs and traditions about childbirth, labor, celebrating this or birthing away from men. If you are an African American woman reading this book, you will have strong ties to your "sisters" in your culture. You may want to have another African American doula working with you at your side. This is great. We hope that you can find such a doula. If you are a birth worker seeking to work with other mothers from a certain culture, we hope you will do so. We hope this short section will help you understand some of the cultures and their birth traditions.

Birth Traditions and Cultural Study:

First, we will start with Mexican birth traditions. This goes back to Aztec times. The father was just as important as the mother in pregnancy and birth because he planted the "seed" of the child. The Aztecs also called Nahua worshipped false "gods" and the conception of a child seemed to be a blessing on the couple from their "gods". The mother could not hide her pregnancy from the community. The family and community would offer a great celebration and feast when they found out the mother was pregnant!

When preparing for labor, the Nahua would make sure the mother was not alone. The midwife was assigned to this mother around when 6 months of pregnancy was left. The midwife would give the mother advice on how to raise her child after birth. So, this was a long-lasting relationship! Also, there were a lot of recommendations for the mother to avoid doing during pregnancy. Today we would consider them a bit superstitious, but the Nahua women took the recommendations seriously. During labor, the mother that was pregnant would become a "warrior" woman. However, in those times it was common for the mother or the baby to die during labor. Sometimes the midwife would help decide who would live. However, many mothers would be prepared for death in order to save her child. The name of the baby was determined by the date and hour of the baby's birth in according to an Aztec calendar.

Another tradition more related to after birth in Latin America is called "La Cuarentena" which means quarantine. So, the mother would go into hiding for around six weeks after birth. The other women of the community would help care for her and her baby postpartum. The mother would abstain from sex, certain foods, and strenuous activities during this time frame.

Another postpartum tradition common to Bali and other areas, the placenta is buried after the baby's birth. This is something I did when I had my baby. My midwife planted the placenta of my daughter under a rosemary bush!

Another tradition in Papua New Guinea is the women would go out into the forest, or somewhere away from the men of the community to give birth. There would be a birthing hut set up. The pregnant mother would labor and give birth in this hut. It was believed the blood from birth was dirty and the men should not touch it. This is why the mother would give birth in such a hut. After labor and delivery, the mother would come back to the community after the birth holding her baby. There are many more cultures one could explore! Do you feel drawn to exploring a particular culture or heritage and birth?

Culture Explore More: Find out more about your culture and birth. If you have a melting pot of cultures from your family tree, then pick one culture that you would like to explore. For instance, if you are African American descent, you may want to explore that culture of birth.

Remember to look for evidence-based articles or at least make sure they have some kind of value to them. We expect you to find at least 3 Internet resources or you may go to your library and find a book about birth traditions as well or purchase one if so desired.

While you are exploring websites about this culture, think of the history of this culture and birth.

Answer these questions:

1. What was this culture's history of birth or postpartum?

2. What is the current present country/culture like today?

3. How do they differ? Do they keep any of the old traditions?

Submit your paper to catholicdoulaprogram@gmail.com

Chapter 7: Anatomy of Birth

We are going to cover a brief overview of the anatomy of a woman and how the baby maneuvers through the birth canal. Some authors call this maneuvering "dancing baby".

Female Body- our "privates":

External female anatomy includes:
Mons pubis
Vulva (which includes the labia, clitoris, urethra, and vaginal opening)
Internal female anatomy includes the:
Vagina
Cervix (this also has an inner and outer area or sometimes called "os" by doctors).
Uterus
Ovaries
Fallopian tubes
Hymen

Bartholin glands and Skene's glands
Female breasts also have external and internal parts.

If you are unfamiliar with the female body, it is best to see a diagram in order to become familiar. We will have a diagram on the next page.

When speaking with a client about her "private" areas – you may want to ask her if she has preferred words like "yoni" to represent the vulva/vagina area. Your client also should be familiar with the definitions of the above words. We want you to write out the definitions of all terms in this chapter and submit it to the instructor. Remember to be sensitive to your client's needs and be respectful when speaking about body parts.

Diagram 1:

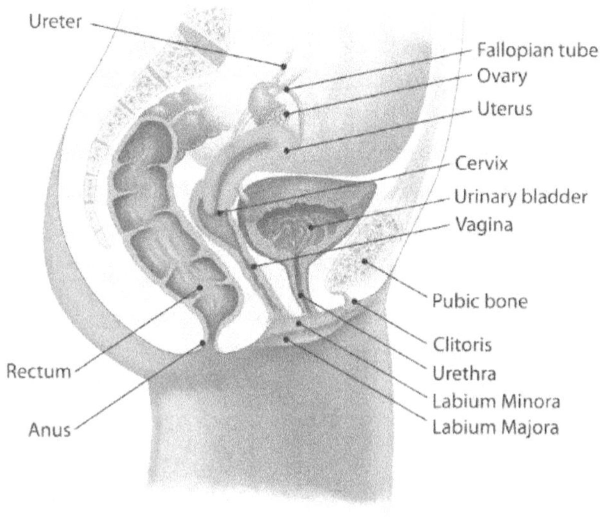

Kocakayaali / Getty Images

This diagram shows the main parts of a woman's insides from ureter – that leads to the uterus to cervix, etc.

Be familiar with the picture as we will have a labeling exercise for students to do for homework or exam assignment. (Please see teacher for the handout to label a similar picture – try not to look – but do it from memory the assignment!)

The vaginal anatomy information[xxix]:

Mons pubis: ***The mons pubis is the rounded, fleshy area on the front of the pelvic bone (the lower belly area) where pubic hair usually grows.***

Labia majora: ***The labia majora are the fleshy outer folds of protective skin located on each side of the vaginal opening. They cover and protect the more delicate external genital organs. "Labia" is the Latin word for lips. The labia majora is often referred to as the outer lips.***

Labia minora: ***The labia minora are skinfolds that are just inside the labia majora. In some people, the labia minora extends past the labia majora.***

Clitoris: ***The clitoris sits at the top of the vulva, above the urethral opening. A fold of skin called the clitoral hood covers most of the***

clitoris, leaving only the tip (nub) visible. The rest of the clitoris is a spongy shaft that goes back several inches inside the body.
<u>Urethral opening:</u> The urethra is the tube that carries urine from the bladder to the outside of the body. Its opening is located below the clitoris, directly above the vaginal opening.
<u>The vaginal opening:</u> The vaginal opening is located between the urethra and the anus.
<u>Bartholin glands:</u> Bartholin glands sit on both sides inside the vaginal opening. They release secretions that lubricate the vagina.
<u>Skene's glands</u>: Skene's glands are located on either side of the urethra. They lubricate the urethral opening. (End of quote).

The Internal Female Anatomy

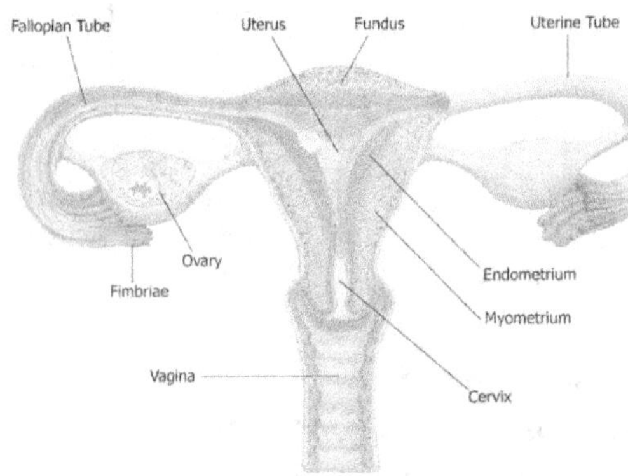

Kinwun / Getty Images

Internal Female Anatomy: Diagram 2: (Note: This will also be another labeling exercise).

Vagina[xxx]: The vagina is a muscular canal that connects the cervix and the uterus. It leads to the outside of the body. Parts of the vagina are made of collagen and elastin, which help it expand during sexual stimulation and childbirth.
Cervix: The cervix is the lower part of the uterus that separates the lower uterus and the vagina. It may play a role in lubrication. While direct contact with the cervix rarely happens during sexual intercourse, some people claim that it helps with sexual pleasure. For others, direct contact with the cervix is painful. During childbirth, the cervix dilates so the baby can move out of the uterus, into the vagina, and out of the body.

Uterus: The uterus is located in the lower belly area between the hips (pelvis), through the vagina just past the cervix. It's also called the womb. The uterus is where a fetus develops during pregnancy. The uterus has three layers of muscle and is one of the strongest muscles in the body.
Ovaries: The ovaries are small organs located on both sides of the pelvis. They play an important role in female hormone production and produce eggs during ovulation.
Fallopian tubes: The fallopian tubes connect the ovaries to the uterus on each side. Hairlike structures called cilia guide the egg from the ovary to the uterus.
Hymen: The hymen is a thin tissue that sits at the vaginal opening. It has no known biological function. The hymen becomes more elastic with age and breaks or ruptures at some point in a person's life.[xxxi]

Female Breast Anatomy: Diagram 3:

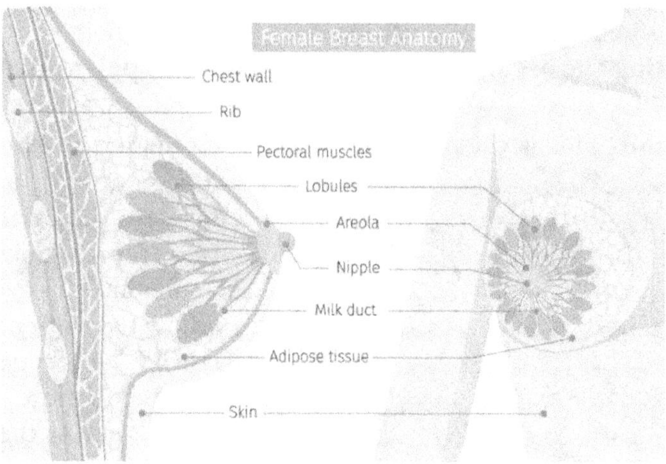

MatoomMi / Getty Images

The breast contains multiple structures within it, including:
Adipose tissue: Each breast has fatty (adipose) tissue that is used to store extra energy.
Lobules: There are 15 to 20 sections called lobules in the fatty tissue. They are attached to ducts that can produce milk.
Milk ducts: The milk ducts are internal structures that go to the areola and nipple, which are the outer portion of the breast.

Areola and nipples: The areola is the darker area on the outside of the breast that surrounds the nipple in the center.[xxxii]
The baby needs to latch onto the areola area as well as the nipple.

(This will also be a labeling exercise). Email instructor for labeling exam.

Types of Pelvis and Uterus Layers:

In this section we will cover types of pelvis and also cover some of the 3 layers of the uterus and functions of why this is important for labor.

"Your pelvis is a group of bones located in the lower part of your torso, between your lower back and your thighs. It has several important functions, including:

***supporting the weight of your upper body**
***acting as a connection point for your lower limbs, as well *as various muscles**
***helping you stand, walk, or run**
***protecting the organs located in or around the pelvic area."**[xxxiii]

"Gynecoid. This is the most common type of pelvis in females and is generally considered to be the typical female pelvis. Its overall shape is round, shallow, and open. Android. This type of pelvis bears more resemblance to the male pelvis. It's narrower than the gynecoid pelvis and is shaped more like a heart or a wedge.

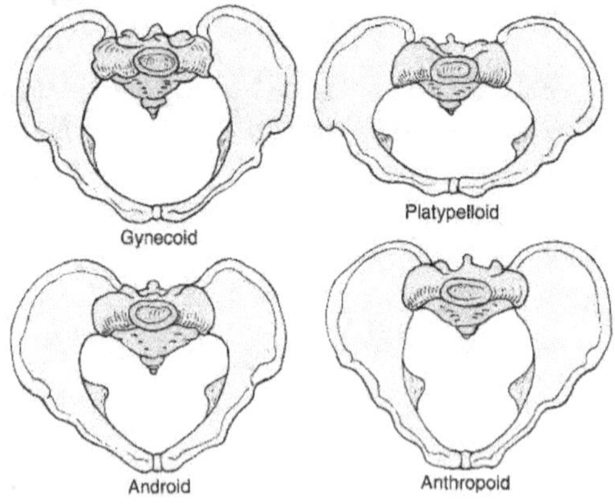

Anthropoid. An anthropoid pelvis is narrow and deep. Its shape is similar to an upright egg or oval.

Platypelloid. The Platypelloid pelvis is also called a flat pelvis. This is the least common type. It's wide but shallow, and it resembles an egg or oval lying on its side."[xxxiv]

Giving Birth based on type of pelvis:

"Now let's talk about how the different types of pelvis shapes can affect childbirth:

Gynecoid. The gynecoid pelvis is thought to be the most favorable pelvis type for a vaginal birth. This is because the wide, open shape gives the baby plenty of room during delivery.

Android. The narrower shape of the android pelvis can make labor difficult because the baby might move more slowly through the birth canal. Some pregnant women with an android pelvis may require a C-section.

Anthropoid. The elongated shape of the anthropoid pelvis makes it roomier from front to back than the android pelvis. But it's still narrower than the gynecoid pelvis. Some pregnant women with this pelvis type may be able to have a vaginal birth, but their labor might last longer.

Platypelloid. The shape of the platypelloid pelvis can make a vaginal birth difficult because the baby may have trouble passing through the pelvic inlet. Many pregnant women with a platypelloid pelvis need to have a C-section."

*Discuss one thing you learned about pelvis types and submit it to your instructor.

How do you know what type of pelvis you have? A regular doctor could take an X-ray, but this is not done as much. If you are going to a midwife, she can usually do something called pelvimetry – she can feel the pelvic bones with her hands and give a good guess at what type of pelvis you have. So, if you can find out it is a plus, otherwise don't worry about it too much. Some groups of women from various cultures also may have one particular pelvis type over another. The Platypelloid pelvis for instance is only in 3% of women and affects Asian or native North Americans the most. Anthropoid pelvis will be more popular for women of African American descent for instance. Also, taller woman with narrow shoulders may have this type. So, you can look for more outward sides as well. The Android pelvis is 30% common among Caucasian women and this type may lead to more cesarean sections or slower labors. The Gynecoid pelvis is the most common type. So, if you are concerned with this, find out what culture your client is from when doing your intake form.

Health conditions that may affect pelvis and be a concern for labor and delivery: Quoted from Healthline article:

> "*Pelvic floor dysfunction.* This is when the muscles of your pelvic floor have trouble coordinating to help you go to the bathroom. It can lead to incontinence and pain in your pelvis or lower back. Pregnancy is a common cause.
>
> *Pelvic organ prolapse.* Prolapse can happen when the muscles of your pelvic floor weaken. As a result, pelvic organs — like your uterus — can drop or even press out of your vagina. Common causes are childbirth, menopause, and aging.
>
> *Sacroiliitis.* Sacroiliitis is when the joint that connects your pelvis to the lower part of your spine becomes inflamed and painful. It can happen during pregnancy or due to an injury or arthritis.
>
> *Osteitis pubis.* Osteitis pubis happens when the joint in the front part of your pelvis becomes inflamed and painful. It's often caused by repeated stress to the area through activities like playing sports.
>
> *Pelvic fractures.* This is when there's a break in one of the bones of your pelvis. Pelvic fractures are often caused by injuries or accidents. Some may require surgery to repair.
>
> *When to talk with a doctor:*
>
> If you're pregnant or planning to become pregnant and have concerns about how your pelvis shape might affect childbirth, speak with your doctor. They can examine your pelvis to help get an idea of how it's structured.

Remember that many other factors besides the shape of your pelvis can affect whether you give birth vaginally. As with the type of pelvis you have, many of these things are out of your control." **<u>End of Quote.</u> Written By Jill Seladi-Schulman, PhD**

Discuss one thing you learned about anatomy on the forum for the class (if taking for credit).

<u>Uterus Section and understanding cycles:</u>

We will now cover the function of the uterus and its role for laboring mother. Quotes are from an article from Cleveland Clinic.

The three main jobs of your uterus are:

Pregnancy: Your uterus stretches to grow your baby during pregnancy. It can also help push your baby out of your vagina.
Fertility: Your uterus is where a fertilized egg (conception or real baby) implants during conception and where your baby grows.
Menstrual cycle: Your uterine lining is where blood and tissue come from during menstruation.

Understanding Menses Cycles:

What happens to your uterus during menstruation?
During your menstrual cycle, the lining of your uterus goes through several changes. The lining (called the endometrial lining) gets thicker and richer with blood as you near ovulation (releasing an egg from the ovaries). If an egg is fertilized during that cycle, it implants into the lining of your uterus, and pregnancy begins.

Your <u>endometrial lining</u> sheds if pregnancy doesn't happen (this is your period). This process repeats every menstrual cycle unless pregnancy occurs.
(<u>https://my.clevelandclinic.org/health/body/22467-uterus</u>).

Isn't the uterus amazing?! Understanding your menses cycles can help you also understand pregnancy and birth too.

What happens to your uterus during pregnancy?

"If conception occurs during your menstrual cycle, the fertilized egg implants into your uterine lining. The fertilized egg (called a blastocyte) burrows into the endometrial lining of your uterus (implantation)." Pregnancy starts at the moment of conception and continues till the baby is born (our comment).

"Your uterus grows and stretches like a balloon to accommodate your growing baby. It contracts during labor and delivery to help push your baby out of your vagina. After about six weeks, your uterus returns to its pre-pregnancy size (although, it can be slightly larger and show signs of being stretched)."

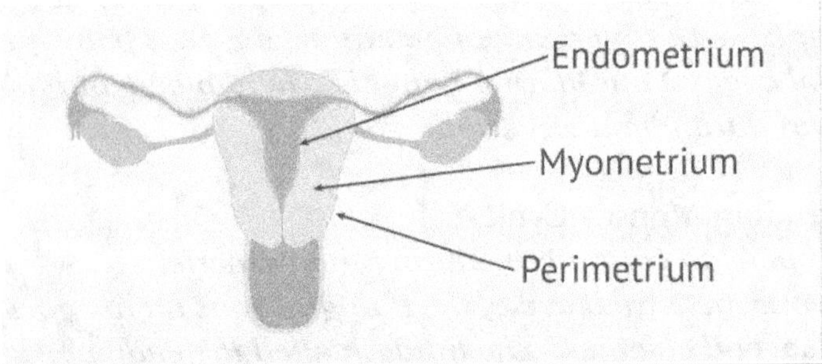

Your uterus consists of three layers:

"Perimetrium: The outermost, protective layer.

Myometrium: The highly muscular middle layer. This is what expands during pregnancy and contracts to push your baby out.

Endometrium: The inner layer or lining of your uterus (uterine lining). This layer of your uterus is shed during your menstrual cycle."

How big is your uterus during pregnancy?

"Your uterus is one of the most unique organs in your body. It can stretch from the size of a lemon to the size of a watermelon during pregnancy. Your uterus can be up to 2 pounds when your baby is born. Your uterus shrinks down to its normal size (a process called involution) and position about six weeks postpartum (after giving birth).

What are the positions of the uterus?

Your uterus can lie in several positions. A typical uterus tilts forward at your cervix and points towards your abdomen. This is called an anteverted uterus. Most people have an anteverted uterus.

If you don't have an anteverted uterus, you might have a:

Retroverted uterus: Commonly called a tipped or tilted uterus. This is when your uterus is tilted or tipped backward so it curves toward your spine instead of forward toward your abdomen.

Anteflexed uterus: Your uterus is anteflexed when it's bent forward. The tilt is severe and can put pressure on your abdomen or bladder and cause painful symptoms.

Retroflexed uterus: Your uterus is retroflexed when it's bent backward. The tilt puts pressure on your lower back."[xxxv]

Anyway, so how does knowing about the uterus help you with labor knowledge? First of all, the myometrium lining of uterus kind of moves around during labor. They help push the baby out so to speak. So, remember this and know that this is part of normal labor for mother to feel contractions and or pressure waves during labor.

*Discuss one thing you learned from the uterus section on the forum.

Cardinal Movements and Labor Anatomy:

One thing, you can watch these short videos to learn about it – but we will also go over some as well.

Video:
https://www.youtube.com/watch?v=q1jmVN3ILpY
Video:
https://www.youtube.com/watch?v=fpBNyecyOzE

What are the Seven Cardinal Movements that babies make during birth?
Engagement
Descent and Flexion
Internal Rotation
Extension
External Rotation
Expulsion

Engagement:

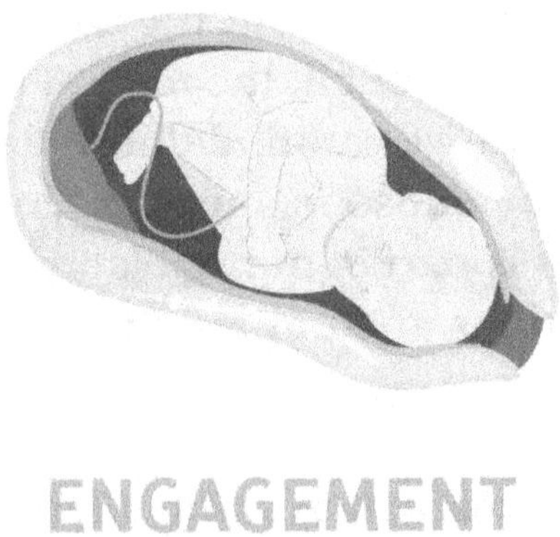

This can happen a few days or weeks before the baby is born. The baby drops into the pelvis more securely and the baby's head has passed into the pelvic inlet. This is almost the start of the labor process. You might also call this engagement a "0" zero in baby station – where the baby is sitting inside the mother. (Our comment – also notice the *fontanel* or head structure of the baby – this is why the baby's head bones do not close up till after birth – they need to be flexible enough to go through the birth canal! Amazing!)

Continuing Seven Cardinal Movements….

Descent & Flexion – these two movements go together:

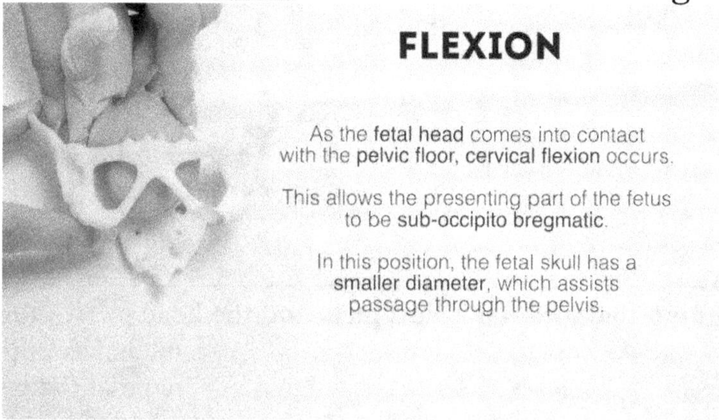

"Descent, sometimes called "lightening", is the movement of your baby's head through the bony part of the pelvis and reaches the depth of the pelvic cavity. As descent happens, flexion is also occurring. During flexion, your baby's head pushes against pelvic tissue, aligning their head with their chin toward their chest."[xxxvi]

Internal Rotation

"Your baby rotates his/her head and body from side to side to front to back to navigate the changing diameters of the pelvis." Our comment: **Think about it – the baby is going through a "dance through the pelvis" in order to be born. No wonder a baby might look beat up after labor and delivery. Sometimes a baby chin gets stuck or does not come out as described. There are baby's that get born "sunny side up!"**

(Our comment – if you do not know some of the definitions in this section -look up the word on a medical dictionary online and add it to your word/term list to turn in for grading at end of course.)

Continuing….Seven Cardinal Movements… Extension

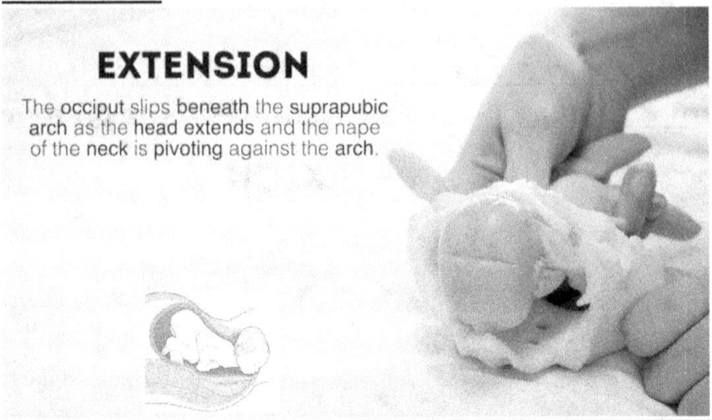

"After internal rotation is complete and the head passes through the pelvis at the nape of the neck, a rest occurs as the neck is under the pubic arch. Extension occurs as the head, face, and chin are born."[xxxvii]

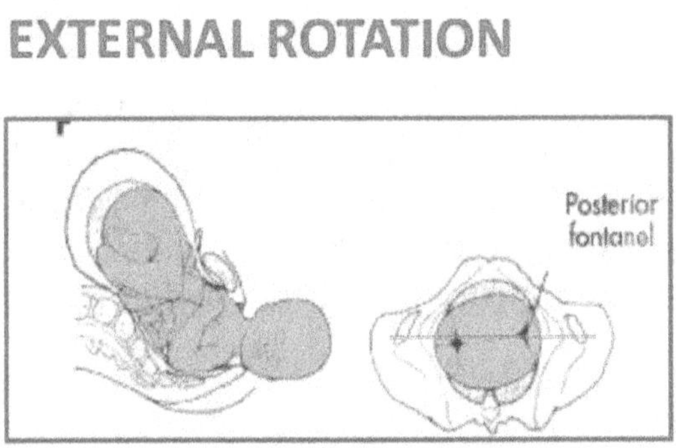

External Rotation

"After the head of your baby is born, there is a slight pause in the action of labor. During this pause, your baby will rotate from face-down to 90 degrees to face towards one of your thighs." (Same resource as above).

Expulsion- or baby is born!

"Your baby's body follows the rotation of the head, and this allows the top and then bottom shoulders to be born!"

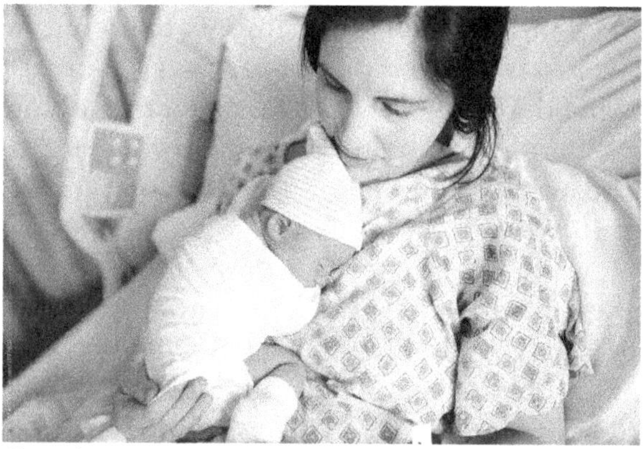

See instructor for labeling and quiz exam over this chapter. For lack of space, we will ask you to email the instructor for this. Thank you. Email comfortinbirth@gmail.com or catholicdoulanews@gmail.com.

Some Extra Anatomy Definitions (From previous *Comfort in Birth Method* book):

Here are some definitions laid out that relate to the mother's stages of labor:

1. Braxton-Hicks Contractions: These are "false labor" contractions that prepare the mother's uterus for labor. They will usually be irregular and can happen at any time of the day.

2. Dilation: 0 centimeters, 1 centimeter, up to 10 centimeters. Abbreviated as usually 1 cm, 2 cm, 3 cm, etc. What does this mean? "This term is in regard to your cervix. Your cervix is a tube-like structure connecting your vaginal canal and your uterus where your baby is. Your baby will pass through your cervix during delivery. As labor approaches, your cervix begins to open preparing to allow your baby out. Dilation refers to how open your

cervix has become. This term will be used in conjuncture with a number in cm. For instance, your doctor may say, "You are 2 cm dilated." This means that your cervix is open 2 cm or about two fingers in width. As a ruler to hold this against when you are in the final stages of your labor and begin to push your cervix will be open or dilated to 10 cm."[xxxviii]

3. Effacement: This is a sister term to dilation that is also in regard to your cervix. As your cervix opens, it will also thin and become shorter. Your doctor may say something like, "You are 1 cm dilated and 20 percent effaced." This would mean your cervix is open one cm, or around one fingers width, and has thinned 20 percent of its original size. Before your baby is delivered your cervix will efface to 100 percent making it paper-thin[xxxix].

4. Soft/Hard Cervix: "Your doctor saying your cervix is firm or hard would simply mean it has not begun to change. If your doctor says your cervix is soft, it means it has begun to prepare for labor.

5. Engaged/Lightening: The term engagement or lightening of your baby means that he or she has dropped further into your pelvis in preparation for delivery. This usually occurs in the last few weeks of your pregnancy. You may notice you breathe easier or your belly changed shape."[xl]
Note: This happened to me on more than one occasion; however, one time the baby dropped so low that it made my back hurt more. So, if a mother tells you the doula that she now can "breathe better, but her back hurts more" – this means the baby has moved down more into the pelvis and is preparing for labor. You can encourage this mother by saying – "Your baby is most likely more engaged now and will be coming soon!"

6. Station: (+1, -2, 0, etc.): "This term is usually used in conjuncture with the term engaged or lightening. Station refers to your baby's position in your womb in reference to two bony spines on your pelvis and can vary from a +3 to a -3. A -3, -2 or -1 station means that your baby has not yet dropped into your pelvis or engaged and is 3-1 cm above the bony spurs in your pelvis depending on the corresponding number. 0 Station means that the baby is level with the bone spurs and has dropped. +3, +2, or +1 mean the baby is 3-1 cm below the bony spurs in your pelvis. Positive stations indicate a move towards the cervix and usually mean labor is imminent."[xli]

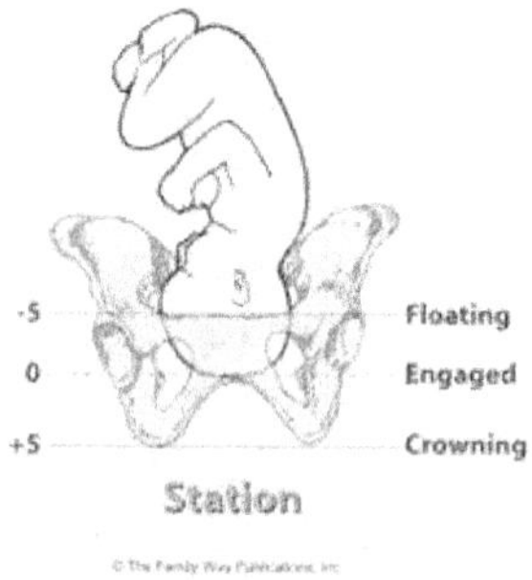

Combining info above we can say: "You are soft 2 cm dilated, 45 percent effaced, and your baby is at -1". This means your cervix is soft or ready for labor, open 2 cms, thinned 45 percent of its original size and your baby is 1 cm above the bones in your pelvis. All of this information is an attempt to estimate when labor will occur.

7. Posterior/Anterior: "These terms refer to the way the baby is facing. This isn't particularly important until during your labor. Posterior means that the baby is facing up with the back of its head against your spine or posterior region, rather than anterior or facing down with the back of the head against your tummy. In a normal labor, a baby faces down making it easier to pass through the birth canal. A baby that is facing posterior can be delivered but may increase the risk of c-section and will result in more back pain for you during delivery."[xlii] – Note we go over more about this in the positions chapter.

8. "Breech position is another term used to describe the position your baby is in. The ideal position for a baby to be in at the time of labor is called vertex position meaning the baby is head down in the uterus. Breech position or breech means that

the baby's feet or butt down rather than head down. When the feet are down and one or both feet will exit the cervix first this is called a footling breech. When the butt is down, but the feet and legs are folded up by the head this is called a frank breech, and finally if the butt and feet are down in almost a kneeling position this is called complete breech." We talk later on about how to get a baby to turn that is breech – but remember this is out of scope of practice of a doula – the mother should consult her doctor or midwife on techniques. Also, a mother can have a natural birth with a breech baby – if a midwife is experienced enough with this – she can help assist that mother. Most regular doctors will only say to have a C-section.

9. "Traverse position, which may just be called traverse, means that the baby is laying sideways or shoulder/arm down towards the cervix. Sadly, traverse positioned babies almost always result in c-section if they can't be turned before labor begins." This is when if you see a hand and no head coming out of the mother that it is definitely time to call 9-1-1 if the midwife has not arrived yet!!

10. Crowning: "Finally crowning, crowing, or crowned means your baby's head is visible to your doctor outside of your vagina during delivery. This means the baby is almost out, and you're almost done."[xliii] Once the baby's head comes out then usually the baby will immediately come out the rest of the way OR there maybe another contraction for the mother to push the rest of the baby out. If the mother is having difficulty – than you may need to look at possibility of shoulder dystocia and the midwife or doctor will need to take care of that situation.

Write down at least three things you learned from this part of the anatomy of birth:

1.
2.
3.

Chapter 8: Understanding Diagnostic tests and Gestational Diabetes

There is a lot to learn about pregnancy and tests and such.

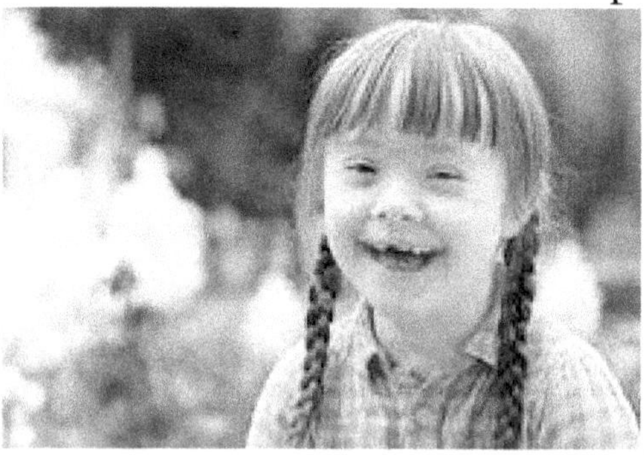

This added on chapter hopes to help you understand tests for mothers a little more. Some tests for mothers are done way before a doula would be hired. However, you might be hired earlier – so a mom may ask you about something. **Certain diagnostic tests are for genetic reasons only**. If a mother is Christian or accepts the child "as is" – there may be no need for these procedures. **For example: A Christian mother will love her child even if "Down Syndrome." However, she may find out other ways like an ultrasound can detect the neck folds of a Down Syndrome child and there may not be any need for amniocentesis for example**. The ultrasound technology now days can show most things that a couple will need to know. However, **if the doctor recommends other tests, make sure the couple knows they have right to refuse unless there is some other reason that seems to be pressing.** Another for instance, I worked with a mother whose baby had a weird heartbeat rhythm. The midwife suggested they go to a perinatal doctor. The doctor did a 3D ultrasound and found out that this was something that would correct itself and no danger to a home birth. The baby's heart returned to normal before the birth and the couple had a wonderful home birth experience. So, we think that a **doctor needs to explain things and let mothers have a right to refuse if so need be**. Some of the tests can cause miscarriages – like amniocentesis. So, this should be decided on very carefully. **Ask the couple if there is anything you can do to help ease their fears of any testing**!

There are a lot of diagnostic tests now for mothers. You will most likely not be asked about them since most of the tests are done way before a mother hires a doula! However, **understanding the types of procedures is important**. See below for list of tests to read about.
Here's an article you can read more about this testing: https://www.hopkinsmedicine.org/health/treatment-tests-and-therapies/amniocentesis
In fact **John Hopkins** also has a list of other common tests: https://www.hopkinsmedicine.org/health/wellness-and-prevention/common-tests-during-pregnancy
These tests can include:
1. Genetic Screening
2. First Trimester
3. Second Trimester
4. Ultrasound
5. Amniocentesis (mentioned)
6. Chorionic Villus sampling
7. Fetal Monitoring
8. Glucose (for diabetes testing)
9. Group B Strep
And others.

We are going to do is give a short sympnosis of a few tests or procedures that doctors usually do in this chapter and give pros/cons for you to guide mothers.

1. ***Abdominal Palpation* (also known as Leopold's Maneuvers). Leopold's Maneuvers is a set way of palpating the uterus to see where the baby is lying down inside the pregnant mother's belly. *What happens*: The mother lies down on a bed and the midwife (usually done more by them) will palpate the uterus to see which**

way the baby is lying at inside the belly. She usually can tell whether baby is head down or head up with this procedure as well. She may also measure the fundus to pubic bone for a week-by-week measurement of the growing baby. Any cons? A mother may not like being pressed on or palpated, but this "procedure" is a good way to tell where the baby is located at in the uterus.

2. *Alpha Feta Protein Test.* This is also known as Maternal Serum Alpha-Feta Protein test. This screening can identify whether a baby has Down Syndrome or if a baby has Trisomy 18 or a baby with neural tube defects – such as spina bifida. It can also diagnose a few other issues like urinary tract, etc. *What happens* – This is a blood test and blood will be drawn out. Concerns or "cons"? There is a 10% false positive rate for this test, so many women maybe scared into an abortion for instance for no reason at all. This test should not be used alone but with other tests. As a Christian mother, it might make more sense not to do such a test because the inaccurate false positives.
3. *Amniocentesis: What happens;* For instance Amniocentesis is more than just a test, it is a procedure where the doctor sticks a needle through the mother's uterus to gain a bit of the amniotic fluid surrounding the baby. The cells are examined in a lab. Tests can take 3 weeks to come back to the parents. It is very accurate for Down syndrome. Test is done around 15 to 18 weeks of pregnancy. *Cons:* However, this test is very invasive and costly. Most women who do it are also at risk for miscarriage (though it is a small risk – it is a risk non the less!) As a Christian mother, I would accept any child born to me – I would personally decline such a test.

4. *Amniotic Fluid Index Test:* This test shows how well the amniotic fluid is being processed by the baby. The baby eats and swallows and pees out amniotic fluid through his or her life in the womb. *What happens*: An ultrasound exam – a pocket of the fluid within the uterus is measured and compared to normal levels. Cons: In late pregnancy this test is not very accurate – as the baby is bigger and a doctor may not catch all levels. Also, if a mother is not drinking enough fluids herself this could cause ratios to be off. Low level fluids are often basis for inductions, but this test alone should not be basis for that.
5. *Chorionic Villis Sampling:* This test is still considered a new procedure. *It examines placental tissue, looking for genetic disorders. Chorionic villi are minute tendrils of tissue that collect the maternal blood as it arrives into the spaces in the placenta. Since tissue from the villi is genetically identical to the fetus – this is one way to find the makeup of the fetus. What happens: The test takes place in hospital and women lies on her back in stirrups. The baby is found on ultrasound and a needle is inserted into the vagina and cervix and a small piece of the fetus' placental tissue is gently suctioned out.*[xliv] Cons: This test is done around 10 weeks after last menses cycle. This is a super early test and seems like it is a little too early. There are other tests like the blood test above (though not always accurate at least it is not as invasive). CVS cannot detect any neural defects. Pros: The CVS might be more reassuring if a family has genetic issues. Cons: The CVS has a higher miscarriage rate than amniocentesis.
6. *Glucose Screening or Glucose Tolerant Test:* We will talk a little bit more about this later – for now these are tests to help determine if the mother has gestational

diabetes or not. What happens: The first test is a screening. She fasts for a few hours and drinks the Glucola drink then the blood test is done. If mother fails it, then she goes to the hospital fasting for several hours (like from night before) and does a harsher screening. Both tests require drinking an awful drink of "Glucola". Cons: The drink can give false positive because a mother may not be used to drinking such sugary nonsense. What can be done instead is discussed below.

7. ***Rhesus Negative Testing;*** If a mother's blood is Rh negative and baby's blood is Rh positive then there is some chances of reactions between mother and baby's blood types. This usually only happens if mother has had a chance to mix blood in past – previous miscarriage, abortion, etc. If father's blood is also negative, then there is no possibility of reaction. What happens: "During the scheduled blood tests, the mother's blood is tested for Rhesus status, and if she is negative and the father's positive, then her blood is tested during the pregnancy for antibodies, and she is given the Rhogam, which prevents sensitization by destroying fetal blood cells in the mother's body."[xlv] Cons: There are some risks for infection because of the nature of this vaccination. A mother may want to consult a more natural minded doctor for alternatives.
8. ***Group B Strep:*** It is a bacterium that is present in about one third of the population. If it is present inside the vagina when giving birth, there is some slight chance of baby getting an infection as well. Most hospitals test for it around 36-37 weeks. What happens: At a routine pregnancy exam, a midwife or doctor will swab the vagina and anus area for containments. They will return with results within a few hours to a day depending on

lab used. If during labor, they can tell mother within minutes if she has this. (Sometimes women are not tested till laboring). What is the "cure"? Well, the medical community likes to give a mother IV antibiotics for this instead of offering natural other alternatives to do. (I had 3 IV antibiotics because of GBS positive – my first baby I didn't need it). Midwives sometimes offer Hibclens – but this is still a type of medicine; but it might help. Hibclens is used on the vagina area per midwife instructions. Another "natural method" can be garlic, oregano or other herbs and probiotics. A mother should consult her midwife or doctor for possible alternatives to the IV antibiotics.

9. ***Ultrasound:*** This is a high frequency sound wave device that can pass into organs such as the uterus. It was discovered by the military! Ultrasound has been used now for awhile to confirm pregnancy, confirm, or change due dates (depending on what doctor sees during an exam), identify the gender of the baby, monitor fetal growth, position of the placenta (to avoid placenta previa), etc. ***What happens:*** A smaller Doppler machine is used for heart rate and such (which works on the sound wave idea but in smaller way). A bigger machine is brought out for actual visual "ultrasound" or also called "sonogram". The woman lies comfortably on a bed or hospital bed. The technician who is trained in this will move around a "wand" over the woman's abdomen with gel to help it glide better. She will take pictures of the inside of what the monitor shows – a baby floating in amniotic fluid. It is a fun experience to see the baby inside the womb. Many times seeing is believing and if any woman who had doubts or thought

about an abortion would “see the veil lifted” inside the womb she will most likely fall in love with her baby! *Concerns of ultrasound:* We do not know enough if “do no harm” is part of ultrasound. Are we harming the infant by putting sound waves at baby developing in the womb? Also diagnosis can still have some inaccuracies – though they are more correct than wrong when it comes to gender for instance. However, the margin of error for weight can be way off up to 15% off. ***Risks include:*** false positive diagnosis of abnormalities, inaccurate gender, inaccurate calendar dates, etc. Also, a mother may have two or more ultrasounds throughout her pregnancy.

10. *Urine Tests:* At most prenatal visits a mother will pee in a cup and the midwife will have a strip to measure things that are going on with the mother’s body. To start out with this is a good way to show if the mother is pregnant to begin with (hormonal HcG will show up). What happens: The mother will pee in a cup at each visit. The woman should provide a mid-stream catch (too early and can be inaccurate results). Concerns: The test will show whether or not what PH scale the mothers urine is supposed to be. For instance, Ketosis or E. coli infection can turn the urine very acidic. Traces of protein or sugar can be issues as well. There are other readings that a doctor or midwife will take from the urine. What a mother can ask: She can ask the midwife to be in charge of the test strip and reading it to her. This makes the mother in charge of her own health and can read her own screenings. I like this approach as it helps the mother feel more in charge of her health care.

Review Question: Write down 3 things you learned about diagnostic tests for pregnancy. What are the reasons the author of the article gave for doing so?

1.

2.

3.

Gestational Diabetes:

Gestational diabetes can be a serious condition during pregnancy. A mother may have to even have insulin if serious enough reasons. A mother will usually be asked to drink some Glucola drink around 20 weeks or so. A mother may even end up with false positives because this drink is super sugary. One thing a mother can do is avoid a lot of starches before the test to get a more accurate reading. There may be other ways to test for gestational diabetes or to go by symptoms. There is controversy in obstetrics about the diagnosis of gestational diabetes and the testing that is done to ascertain which women are at greatest risk. Dr. Michel Odent wrote an article about gestational diabetes: http://www.gentlebirth.org/archives/gdmodent.html

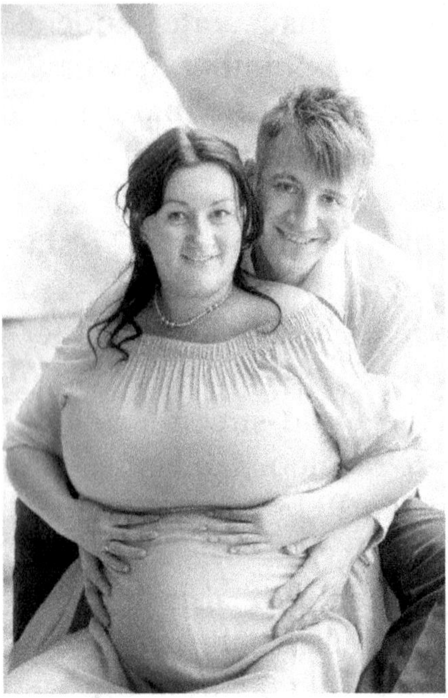

Until all the controversy is resolved and a more scientific test can be offered, we are stuck with the glucose tolerance test at 28 weeks gestational age. The mother can look at the list of who is at greatest risk and decide to decline the test if her risk is low.

A mother can also try the jellybean test as a way to help her know if she has GD or not. Read this article to find out more: https://marionwomenshealthcenter.com/docs/1-hour-jelly-bean-test/ She may need to obtain permission from her doctor. Another way to do testing is like a diabetic – take blood level before and after eating and see where's she at on her glucose levels. She will need a special glucometer to do that kind of testing.
Gloria Lemay article[xlvi]:

Women at risk for Gestational Diabetes:
– maternal age over 25
– – obese woman prior to pregnancy
– – previous birth of baby weighing over 10# at birth
– – previous unexplained stillbirth at term
– – family history of diabetes (esp. close relatives who became diabetic at a young age
i.e. juvenile onset diabetes)
–previous history of recurrent miscarriages
–extremes of heaviness or thinness
–history of alcohol abuse
–history of anorexia or bulimia

This risk factor screening will only pick up 50% of women who are GD. Therefore, we would be wise to treat everybody "as if" they are GD because diet and lifestyle changes are good for everyone (preventive health care).

If your client has any of the above factors, urge her to follow a GD diet and exercise program as early as possible and then, if she does take the 28-week test, she will usually sail through it with flying colors. This does not mean that she can start eating junk food though. I tell my clients that ice cream and chocolate are toxic to unborn babies–there is way too much fat, salt, sugar, and caffeine in these products for a baby in utero to cope with.

Whole, organic foods, fresh water, and love are the ingredients to grow a healthy baby.

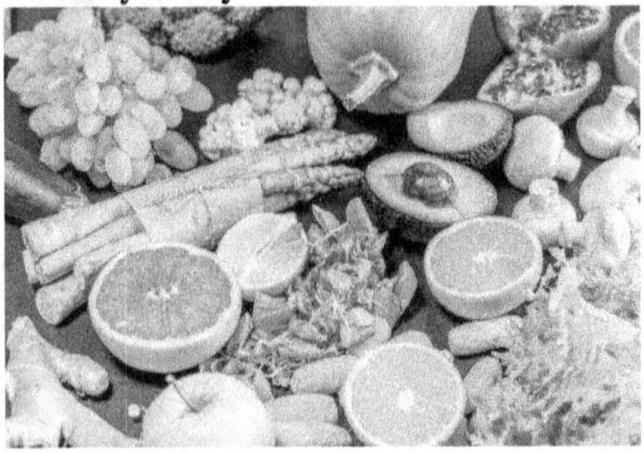

How can we best serve the health interests of mother and baby? If you meet your client prior to the 28-week test, you can let her know that she can improve her chances of passing the test by eating healthy, unrefined food for the week preceding the test and exercising every day (a 20-minute brisk walk that elevates her heart rate). You can explain to her that some healthy women who just ate badly (lots of sweet desserts and junk food) prior to the 28-week test have tested positive for risk of GD and then had to undergo the more unpleasant fasting 3-hour blood tests.

If you meet your client after she has been diagnosed as GDM (gestational diabetic mother), I encourage you to attend with your client at the diabetic clinic where a nurse will give her counseling and nutrition advice. Usually, the woman will be asked to maintain a food diary and daily 'exercise after meals' regimen. She will be shown how to test her own blood and may be asked to count the number of times her baby kicks in a 12-hour period. The philosophy behind the diet is that the GDM needs to control her blood sugar levels at an even rate (also known as staying in the Zone–not getting stuffed or starved) and can do so by "grazing" on small amounts of wholesome food, eaten often.

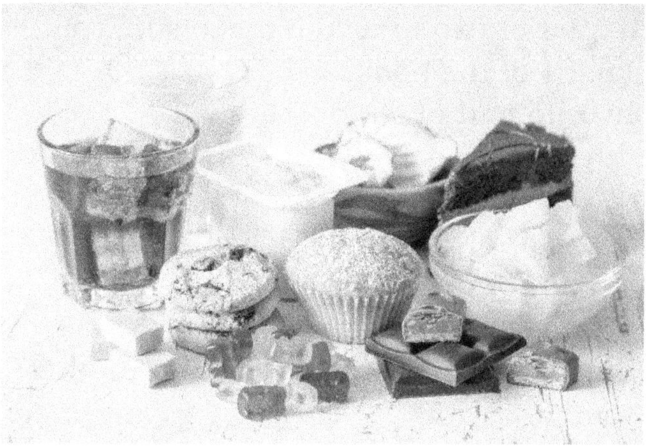

Gloria LeMay: "What foods should your clients avoid?
*sugar (white or brown)
*honey, molasses, syrup, jams, jellies, marmalade
*chocolate, candy
*puddings, Jell-O, fruit yogurts
*desserts—cakes, pies, pastries, iced cookies, etc.
*soft drinks, tonic water
*sweetened condensed milk
*sweet sauces—oyster sauce, teriyaki, plum, sweet & sour, ketchup

Caffeine has been shown to make the body more resistant to the effects of insulin so tea, coffee and all soda pop should be avoided. Fruit sugar should only be consumed in small portions. ½ a banana, 10 grapes, a small apple are the serving sizes. Milk products are also high in sugar and should be used in moderation according to the advice of a **diabetic nutritionist."**[xlvii] **End of article by Gloria LeMay**

If you are not familiar with a gestational diabetes diet, there's a book called "Real Food for Gestational Diabetes" by Lily Nichols. And there's a more general book titled "The Real Food for Pregnancy" which is basis for the Academy of Natural Birth or Kitchen Nutritional Doula™ class.
https://nutritional-doula.thinkific.com/
You may want to choose one of these two books for your book reviews.

Talking about book reviews – guidelines include:

1. **Author/title of book/your name – top of page**

2. Summary of the book in around 500 words or so – choose your favorite chapter or two to read – make sure you choose a little bit of all parts of the book.
3. What was your favorite part of the book?
4. Did you agree with author on everything? If not, why not?
5. Do you think you can apply this book to your doula work? If so, how will you do so?
6. Give the book an "amazon" review.
7. Would you recommend this book to a pregnant mother?
Submit your reviews to your instructor! comfortinbirth@gmail.com

Hyperemesis Gravidium: Severe pregnancy issue…
This section is written not to scare any mother, but to inform. If you are a mother and want to skip reading this – that is fine! This is another serious condition that can happen super early in pregnancy. **Definition of this problem**: **"Want to understand more about Hyperemesis Gravidarum or HG? HG is defined as a potentially life-threatening pregnancy disease that may cause weight loss, malnutrition, dehydration, and debility due to severe nausea and/or vomiting and may cause long-term health issues for mother and baby(ies)."**[xlviii] If a mother has any of these symptoms, she should talk to her doctor immediately. This is not a time to pretend as this is out of scope of practice for a doula. https://www.hyperemesis.org/get-help-now/ Send mom to this link for immediate help. There are also support groups: https://www.hyperemesis.org/who-we-help/family-friends/support-for-mothers-families A doula can start up a support network to help mothers with this disease as it might be called.
Go to www.catholicpostpartum.com to learn more about support for pregnant and postpartum mothers.

Anemic and pregnancy: Some mothers can become anemic during pregnancy. There is usually a time around mid-pregnancy where the midwife will check for blood and hemoglobin count. The numbers should stay around 10-11 for birth. If not, the mother may need to add iron supplementation. The problem with iron supplements is they all cause constipation in mothers. So, if mother can do the following:

*Eat more red meat – with no calcium items (no dairy)**

***Eat more leafy vegetables that have iron in them (spinach, etc.)**

***Eat calcium foods when she is not eating iron – for better absorption.**

*If taking iron supplements, look whole foods supplements – this usually works better – however, many doctors/midwives will insist on their kind – the mother may have to conform to the doctor's wishes – however, this can be an alternative. Standard Process supplements are also considered "nutritional" and are exceptionally great too. Standard Process are usually only available through a chiropractor or other registered physician or naturopathic doctor.

***Note: We are not giving any medical advice here and a mother should always check with her doctor or midwife before taking ANY supplements. Thank you.**

***As a doula may check in with mother to see if she is eating right and taking her supplements. You can encourage her. Also, suggest eating things that will help get her bowels moving (fibrous foods) and drinking plenty of water.**

***Remember as doulas – we are participants in mother's health, but we are not a doctor and we do not diagnose, treat or cure an illness or disease. If a mother has GD, make sure she is following her doctor's directions and or midwives' instructions. She should not be asking you for medical advice.**

You can give her information and let her decide what do to for her health!

Email instructor for quiz over this chapter – email catholicdoulanews@gmail.com or comfortinbirth@gmail.com

Assignment: Make a flier up about Gestational Diabetes for a client – think of 3 tips that could help a mother prevent it.

CHAPTER 9: Stages of Labor and some positions of labor:

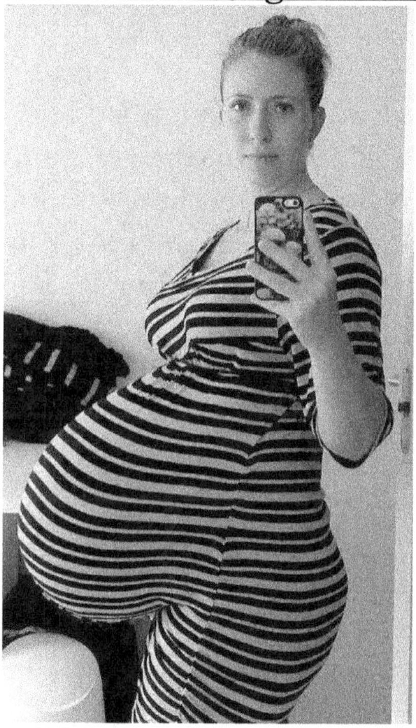

In this chapter we discuss various stages of labor and we do cover some "positioning" as well (even though we have another chapter on that).

I originally wrote about stages of labor as 3 main stages which is the "medical" definition. However, some books continue to add in more stages of labor – so the second part has more defined on how labor can progress in a way that might make more sense. You can also read this linked article below about stages of labor:

https://injoyhealtheducation.com/media/wysiwyg/pdfs/guidesandhandouts/StagesofLabor3-FacilitatorsGuide-English.pdf

The original version of this book – I wrote the following about stages of labor – after that will be an extended version:

> Defining the First Stage of Labor:
> The first stage is usually a preparatory stage. The mother's body may or may not feel surges at this stage. If you go back to the emotions of labor, the stages of labor kind of go along with the emotional stages too. In my second child's birth, I thought I was feeling some labor surges the day before his birth. At the time, I

thought I was in labor! We headed over to the hospital. I was monitored for a while. We discussed my birth plan with the head nurse. However, maybe she scared me a way a bit. She was like "well, you may have this plan, but we do things our way here." For whatever reason, my body just kind of stopped progressing and I was not going to have the baby that day. I ended up going home very hungry and we ate supper at a friend's house! She happened to be my babysitter for my youngest. The following day, my labor started up again with my water breaking! I had my baby without too many issues as I ended up with the night staff that was more interested in helping me birth the way I wanted to.

<u>The first stage of labor</u> is usually around this 0cm-4cm time frame of looking at this from a doctor's perspective. The labor may come and go as mentioned above.
The second part of the <u>first stage</u> of the mother is getting excited and then she is moving to the concentration stage of emotions. The labor surges are becoming stronger. The baby is moving down more and will probably be going from a -2 station to a 0 or further down; the mother's dilation will be around 4 centimeters now. The mother is opening up more and she will probably be setting a better rhythm now. She will be feeling contractions (surges) every five to four minutes. This is the usual time when doctors advise a mother to get to the hospital. However, a mother could stay a little longer at home safely up to even three-minute intervals if she does not need any particular interventions and would like to go to the hospital pushing out the baby. So, if a mother is concerned about hospital germs and

such, we would advise her to stay at home a bit longer if possible.

The ***traditional second stage*** is when the mother goes into transition of the birth. The mother sometimes experiences that feeling of not being able to go on as mentioned in emotions of labor section. The transition stage also can be a peaceful time before pushing. It varies depending on the mother. The pushing stage is the final part of the "third stage" as the mother pushes the baby out, the miracle of birth occurs when the baby arrives! Each time you experience birth as a doula, you will feel this wonderful awesome delight and see the efforts of the laboring mother. (Even if she does have an epidural). The baby is here, and the mother is an awesome "warrior."

The third stage of labor is defined as the placenta being "born" and expulsed from the uterus. The placenta is an amazing organ that many do not contemplate. If one is interested in learning more about placentas, we do encourage you to explore them. Some mothers like to

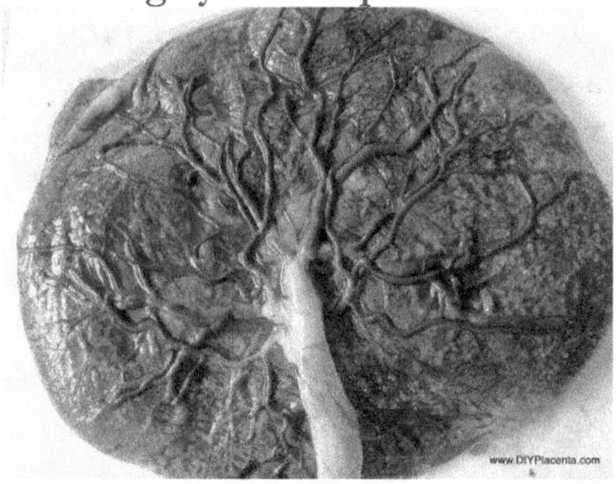

give birth to the placenta and have the cord attached still to the infant baby. This is called "lotus birth." Lotus birth is a way honoring this extra organ. The placenta maybe preserved in herbs or essential oils after birth. The mother will wait for the cord to fall off the baby naturally in most lotus birth traditions. Though a mother could choose a partial lotus where the cord is burned off after the birth of the placenta.

Upright and Active birth:

Many doctors do not allow mothers to birth in an upright position which is better for receiving your baby (mama) or for the mother to receive her baby (doula reading this). So, what is a mama to do? Or a doula to do? As "advocate", we need to ask or even demand that the client receives the best gravity for her birth time. There is an older book titled "New Active Birth" that goes over some tips and techniques for upright positioning. We also can cover some of the ideas and our own ideas in this upright or active birth.

Upright birth or active birth can be accomplished during labor by some of these tips:

Stay active at home as long as possible. Being upright in your home, walking, doing "daily tasks" even while having contractions is what our ancestors did (see history of birth). Once you arrive at the hospital (or client arrives), make sure you tell staff what kind of birth you want – that you want an active birth with little or no interventions – ability to walk the hospital hallways if need be or be on a birth ball upright. I remember one of my labors, I was able to walk the hallways. I ended up going home as the baby was not ready to come down that day; I ended up having my water break at home the next day and going back to hospital to give birth within

4 hours! Walking before labor also can help get labor started!

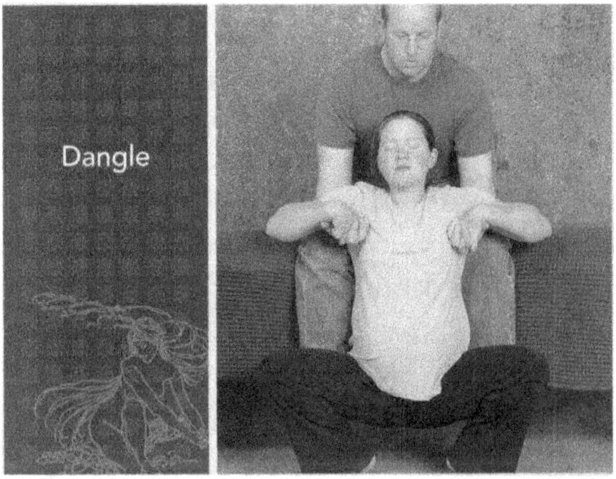

Make sure if you are going to have an IV's or attachments that you can get on a birth ball during labor or sit upright in bed as much as possible. Even trying dangling during pushing can help. As a doula advocate, you should make sure your client's needs are heard. If a client can communicate what she wants before labor starts, then things will go much smoother. I can give an example – one of my clients wanted a water birth. Her second baby was a water birth and she had it all planned ahead of time. Then, she had a third baby, well there was lack of communication about the water birth and she did not get it because of this lack of communication. Communicating beforehand can be the best way to receive and have the active birth you desire (or your client desires)!

One good way for a better and calmer birth is having good preparation for birth. Preparing for birth includes good nutrition (we are relocating to this section below for print edition), good exercise techniques, and good communication with the mother's "birth team".

Expanded edition of this:

First Stage of Labor:

Braxton hicks' contractions are not real labor – but they may prepare mother for real labor. They are preparatory and can last a few weeks before birth.

Some mothers will not feel the first stage of labor that much. In fact, this can even be going on for a few days. It depends on your definition of the first stage of labor. If you go by defining it as 1 cm to 2 cm dilatation, some mothers can be this a week or so before real active labor.

However, others may call this Braxton Hicks contractions – which are more like "practice" for labor and they have no real way to measure. They are not consistent and can go on weeks before a real baby is born. So, for our purposes the first stage of low active labor – the mother will notice something different and she maybe able to go along with her normal activity for a day or two before the more active labor begins.

However, this low active labor will be steadily progressing. Example: I had some contractions and such the day before my son's birth; at the time I did not know when he was going to be born. I went to the hospital even; but I was not progressing that much. They sent me home. Well, the very next day, my water broke and then my labor was really "active". So, I basically had a low-level labor beforehand. So, let us just say sometimes labor begins before you know it and other times it does not.

The first part of *real labor* is *active labor* is usually when the mother will start having progressing contractions and her cervix will be dilated around 4 cm or more. She will be ready to get over to the hospital or call the midwife if having a home birth. If she is going to a birth center, she will most likely call over to find out when the midwife wants her to arrive. She may have contractions that follow the 5-1-1 rule (see below for more definition on this). The mother may have the emotions of feeling excited at this time. Once she gets to more of a concentration stage of emotions, she is now in the later part of active labor (some may call a third part of active labor).

If a mother is in the *concentration stage emotionally* – this will be further into the stage one of labor or active labor; she is most likely already heading to the hospital or have arrived. She wants to have her own space and time to concentrate on labor "waves" or "surges". She may not be as talkative. She will feel the baby progressing downwards towards the pushing time. This also might be called "transition stage". The transition stage is usually the time where the mother is in between Stage One (Active labor) and Stage Two: *time to push the baby out.* Transition stage can last a long time or be short – it depends on the mothers. Some mothers may not even realize they were in transition until the birth happened and they will reflect that "such and such time" was transition for them. It also can be measured around 7 cm to 8 cm or so just before the woman's body is open all the way – however, some women may have transition after 10 cm where they may have a cervical lip (baby's head not ready to come down all the way). So, if the doctor says there is a cervical lip, the mother may need more patience during this time and support.

Read more about cervical lip[xlix] here: https://www.bellybelly.com.au/birth/what-is-a-cervical-lip-how-can-it-hijack-your-birth/

And here: https://www.spinningbabies.com/cervical-lip-solutions/

The mother may want to try different positioning if the baby is not going over this lip. The spinning babies site shows a mother going slightly upside down for a minute. So, we suggest looking at these websites if the mother has this issue. Also, the mother may want to practice a lunge technique if baby's head is not quite down all the way into the pelvis. (This happened to me in my water birth; once I did the lunges – he came on down!)

Second Stage or Pushing Baby out

Now that the baby is coming down and his head is showing – it is time for mother to push baby out. Sometimes, the mother may feel a "ring of fire" as the baby head emerges. This is a natural feeling and just keep encouraging mother that she is "doing a good job" – if you "feel the burn – then your baby is almost here." However, the mother may need to watch out for those shoulders! Sometimes, the baby can get stuck because of shoulder dystocia. https://www.spinningbabies.com/product/free-resolving-shoulder-dystocia-preview/

There is something also called the Gaskin Maneuver to help with shoulders. Here's an article from Midwifery Today about this: https://midwiferytoday.com/mt-articles/flipflop-four-steps-remember/

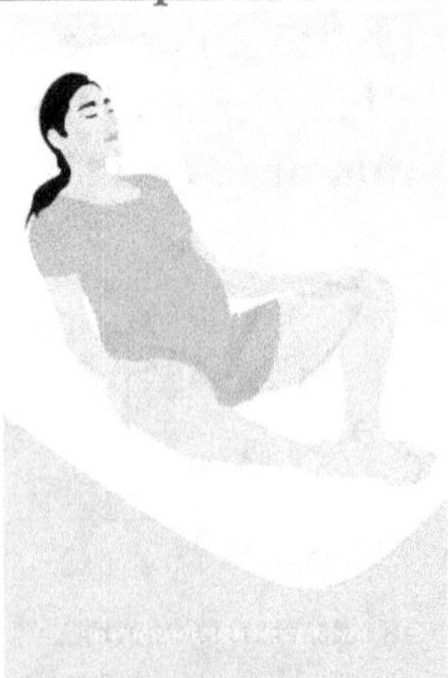

Remember the *doctor would be doing this as this is not in the practice of a doula;* but you may want to know if the doctor or midwife is knowledgeable in this area. https://www.birthinjuryguide.org/birth-injury/types/infant-shoulder-dystocia/ (Another article to read).

Pushing baby out[1] – the best way is an upright position. Gravity works best for baby and mother if momma is more upright position or on hands/knees. Two of my births – I was basically hands and knees – my homebirth and my water birth in hospital. So, what is most common for birthing in hospital?

Usually at the hospital, they will have you sit in a semi-circle position or basically on your back and put your feet in stirrups. Then, they will do the breathing where they count for you or *directed pushing*: "Breathe in one, two, three, four, and five push out....six, seven, eight, nine, ten." This position is not ideal as the baby can get stuck under the mother's bones or mom may end up with the cervical lip situation. Directed pushing is a very common technique for labor.

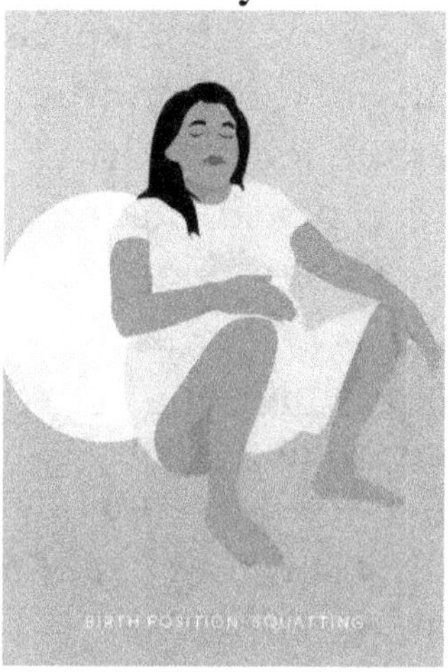

The next position that is better for a mother during labor is to be in a ***squatting position***. Her baby can basically fall down with gravity. The mother will be more relaxed in a squatting position. She also can listen to her body pushing and breathing. She does not have to count and breathe. She can allow her body to relax and breathe out baby naturally or natural pushing. A mom can try natural breathing and pushing in any position. We should encourage her to listen to her body. My water birth, I used the blowing technique in between contractions to open up my lips and to relax – this helped get my baby out. His head came out on one contraction and then second contraction his head popped out along with rest of his body. It was a beautiful birth by listening to my own body and not

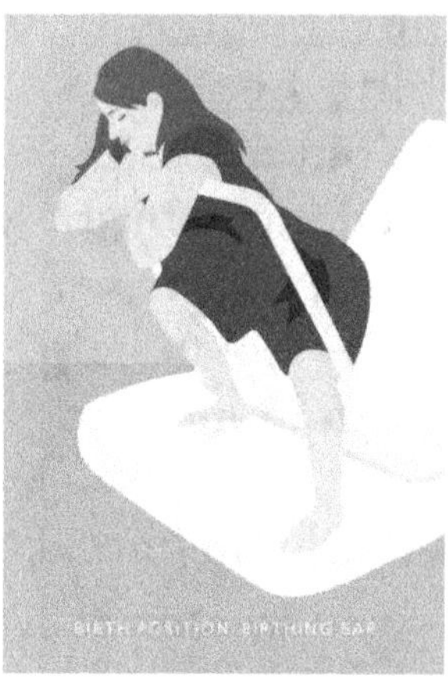

being guided by the hospital staff as much – they only told me to "blow!"

Other positions are possible during labor, you can use a labor bar on the hospital bed – I did not really know about this bar in my births – learned about it later on. I think the hospital staff does not even know that much about it. So, it is important for a mother to be informed that this is possible for her birth. Looking at the above picture – the mother can possibly squat using the bar or at least have something else to hang onto for her birth.

A rebozo can also be used to help with pushing out baby. A Rebozo can be hung from a door or ceiling to help with

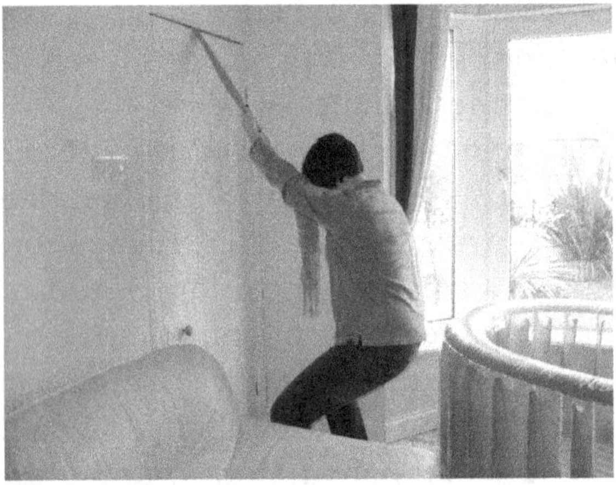

pushing the baby out – this is more ideal for a home birth for instance. (See picture above of rebozo and door). The last one pushing position is the birth stool. I found out that the hospital had a birth stool and they never ever offered it to me. I would have accepted that stool to help push my son out and I probably would have been more relaxed and done sooner!

A mother should be informed about this option to have a birth stool.

There are different types:

http://www.kayabirth.com/

https://www.cubmama.com/

Also, there are some birth stools made out of wood too.

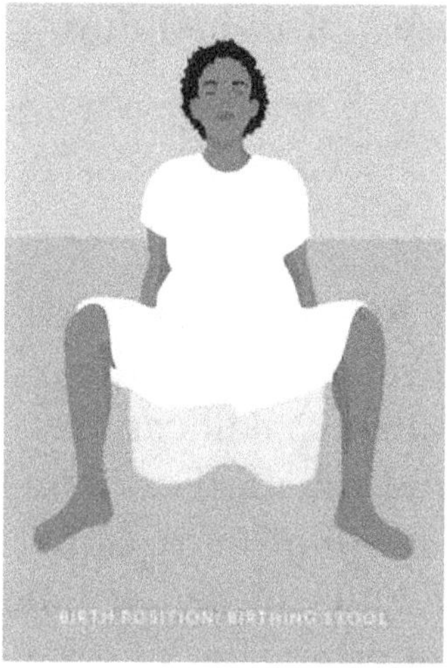

Also, squatting can be considered the ancient way of pushing out a baby. In Africa, a woman is supported by her family, and she goes into a private area to have her baby. Once the baby is born, she only rests for like a day. Then, she is out doing things again like "nothing happened!" Pretty amazing! However, more cultures honor the idea of having a 40-day rest period after birthing. There is a book titled "The First 40 days" which can be another idea for a book review.

Enrichment Assignment D:

Learning about the stages of labor and the placenta are important for birth workers.
First of all, make a small handout or flier about the stages of labor. Include any terms you learned from the term study above. Second, explore more about lotus birth.
Make another flier or handout about lotus birth practices. Try to include at least two internet articles for the above handouts. (Put article resources at bottom of flier or back of flier). Please submit to Comfort Birth Method instructor.

Any questions? Please contact the instructor if taking this class for certification!

Research assignment: Find out what your hospital locally offers in way of birth bar or birth stool or a birth ball for labor and delivery? Can a mother choose to push baby out using a birth stool or birth bar? Can a mother use a birth ball during labor? Can she use a peanut ball?

Submit to instructor.

Birth Ball for Laboring:

A birth ball is a ball a mom can use to bounce on or sit on during labor to help her during labor. Also, a peanut ball can be used for an epidural mother or one confined to bed for other reasons.

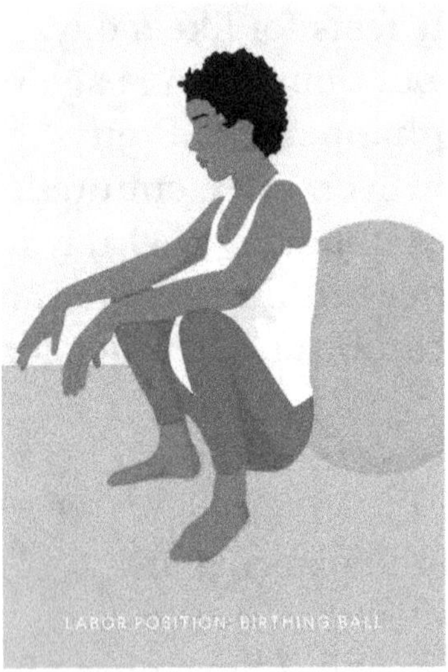

The birth ball can be used along with rebozo together if so desired. We cover more about birth ball in our rebozo level B class. Please ask to enroll in level A and B if you would like more hands-on work and know how.

Assignment: Research on your own:

What are the benefits of using a birth ball or peanut ball during labor?

Write down and submit to instructor what you found. Please submit source.

Sources for our images for this section can be found here: https://www.thebump.com/a/birthing-positions

Email us for quiz over this chapter – email comfortinbirth@gmail.com or catholicdoulanews@gmail.com

Bonus Section: The 3 R's of Labor – Reference to Penny Simkin: 1. **Relaxation**: If a mother is not that relaxed during labor – she is going to have a harder time pushing baby out.

2. **Rhythm:** Once a mother finds her rhythm of birth – this is kind of a combo of things – focusing, staying breathing well during each contraction, and having support person with her – she will most likely stay in a good rhythm. She may lose rhythm when she loses concentration or other factors. This is why a doula is so important.

3. Ritual: Some mothers may have rituals based on cultural or other aspects of labor. Like a Jewish mother cannot have her husband touch her as this is a ritual for them. So, respect other cultures and their rituals. You may want to find out before the birth if there is a ritual expected of you during the birth or afterwards! Some birth rituals go more into after birth and naming the baby, etc.

Role of the partner:

1. Make sure the mother has her support partner: husband, boyfriend, girlfriend, etc. Whoever she wants there to support her during this birth if possible. We know with covid times there are more restrictions; however, you maybe at a home birth where there are less restrictions. Remember to include the partner as much as possible.
2. **Ask the partner:** "Would you like to help her push? Would you like to help wrap the rebozo around mom? Would you like to cut the cord?"
3. **The partner** should be one of the first to help announce gender (if unknown beforehand) to the mother!
4. **Remember as a doula,** the partner plays an important role – ask partner before birth ways they want to participate

or allowed to by their rituals. If the dad is now allowed to touch – still include him and his name as he watches the birth for instance.

5. **Penny Simkin** goes over the 3 R's a lot in her website. We suggest going to www.pennysimkin.com and search through her library of materials to gain more information if so desired. She also uses a technique called "Take Charge Routine" if a mother loses concentration during labor, this routine helps the mother gain concentration back!

*Email instructor for quiz over chapter.

CHAPTER 10: CHOICES AT BIRTH

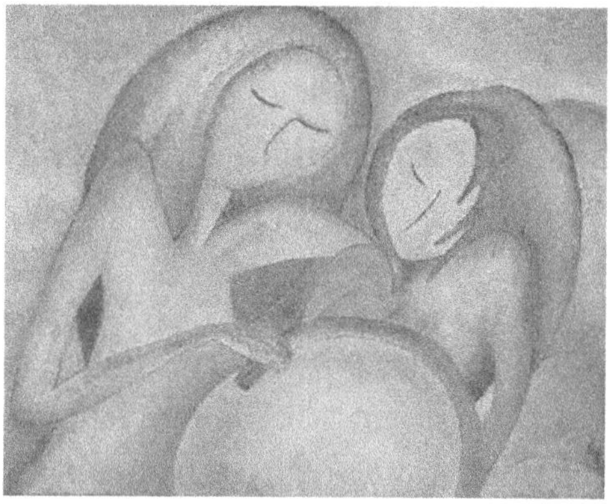

Birth Choices are important for most mothers; however, many mothers are in the hospital birth "trap". We are just calling it a trap because this is the modern way of birth and most women feel that they have no options once they arrive at the hospital. "I must obey my doctor." However, our Comfort in Birth Method™ model we accept the fact that the majority of births are at the hospital, and we as Comfort in Birth™ doulas can help mothers achieve a relaxed, calm, and comforting birth in the hospital. There is a book titled "Homebirth in the hospital" that you may want to read for a book review. Also, the idea of Comfort in Birth™ is to offer the best birth possible to any mother anywhere.* The idea that you cannot have a peaceful birth at a hospital is not true. I had a great water birth experience at the hospital (as I mentioned earlier in this booklet).

*__I wrote most of this book before the covid-19 scare. So, today's hospital practices are definitely different. Most hospitals will require covid-19 testing of the mother. We strongly suggest if you are going to go to hospital – get pre-tested before going into labor if this is what your hospital requires. That will save you some headaches. If you are not tested ahead of time, the baby may be taken away from you without your consent__. Sometimes even the dad or father is not allowed to be there. Something to consider I do not even know if saying **"I do not consent" will make a difference** – but that is something you as a mother may want to consider. Hey, threaten the hospital with a lawsuit if you have to get your point across.

Now that supposedly this 'scare' is under control – the best thing to do is check to see what the hospital policies are like now for your area.

Doulas reading this: **Going to hospital births may involve some restrictions, make sure you check to see how many visitors the hospital allows – do they count doulas as an extra person? Do you need to show a certificate of certification? Do they want you to wear a mask? Etc.**

Virtual doula work can also be an option or offer hybrid – virtual and in person when possible.

<u>Example of OB Care Vs. Midwifery Care:</u>

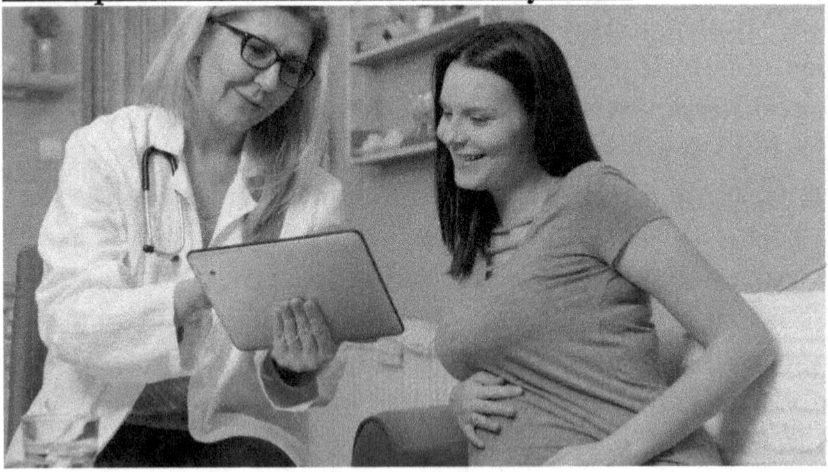

Most mothers you are going to meet with will be having the "normal" birth with an OB/GYN and the mom will most likely be delivering at the hospital nearby – but some

exceptions on hospital location! Some mothers might prefer the "hospital downtown" vs. more local.

What does an OB/GYN do to at a prenatal appointment? Most of the time a mother will go into a doctor's office wait for a half an hour (or longer) to see the doctor and usually there is waiting inside the room! So, once she sees the doctor for like 15 minutes or less, then that's it. The OB moves on to the next patient. There's lack of personal care for most part with OB/GYN. You might stay longer the first visit, but you will be mostly talking to the nurses and not the main doctor!

Now there may be some doctors that spend longer; but the average time with a client is going to be 15 minutes.

Is Homebirth safe? Short answer Yes!

Imagine having a baby safe at home with your local midwife and husband supporting you. You might have a doula present as well. This is the ideal situation for any birth. Why do most women have a baby in the hospital?

Usually, most women have no other option than to have a baby in hospital; they are not familiar with homebirth. Or they may have heard about it; but have decided that it is too risky. Read this article: http://www.naturalbirthandbabycare.com/home-birth/

Research Assignment: Research the safety of homebirth on the Internet – find 3 things you learned from an article and submit to teacher.

What is a midwife like?[li]

I personally was spoiled by our first midwife. We lived in New Mexico out in the "country" and our midwife just happened to live up the road from us!! (What a nice deal!) She would actually come over to our house for all the prenatals – really nice. We had lots of time to talk. Our first appointment was probably like 2 hours or so! The next appointments were at least 20-30 minutes. We had measurements of the baby on the bed, blood pressure, listened to the heartbeat, etc. It was so wonderful to have her come over when she was supposed to (weekly towards the end!)

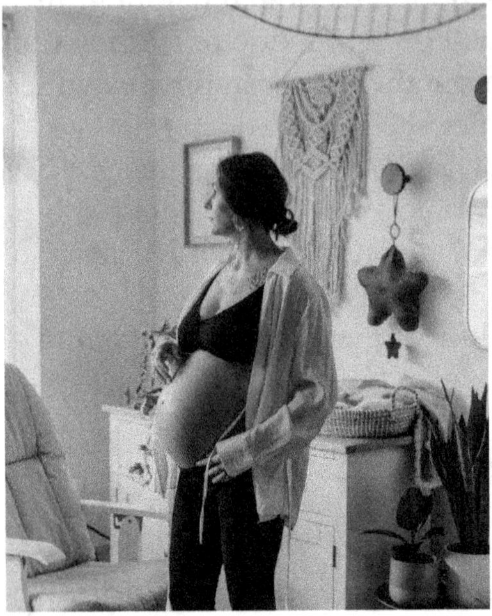

We even could call her in the middle of the night for questions if something happened. One day I had false labor, but it ended up stopping – she gave us some good advice (like if you had been not doing much – get up and move around take a shower, etc.) So, a midwife spends a lot of personal care time with you! Even if you have to go to her office, it is worth the trip. Some midwives will still come to you as well. Depends on the midwife! A birth center midwife is similar to above; but you go to her birth center for the prenatals and have the baby at the birth center.

Question: If you are a mother reading through this: Have you ever experienced a homebirth, hospital birth or birth center birth? What was it like?

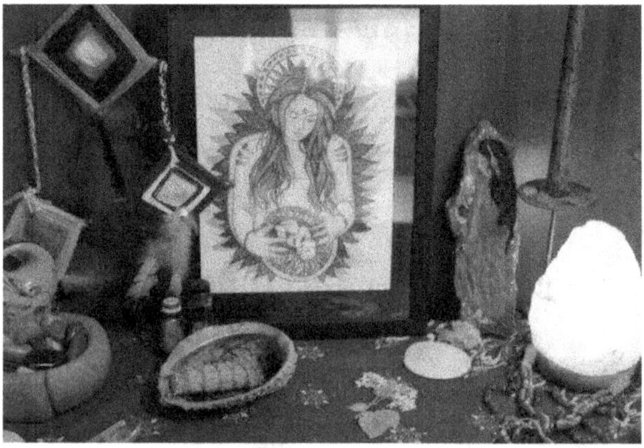

A Sacred Space for birth[lii] to occur may include:

*Keeping the lights low for mother

*Ensuring less "traffic" in a hospital room.

*Keeping quietness in the room as much as possible.

*Keeping mother calm and relaxed.

*Light music in background (if mother chooses).

*Have a religious picture for "focus".

*Being the mother's advocate.

*Keeping the mother CALM during labor.

*Having an atmosphere that is sacred.

*Honoring the laboring mother "groaning cake" – this is sometimes made during childbirth by various cultures.

*Knowing when to touch or not touch the mother. Some mothers may prefer you to be present at birth, but not to touch. A mother may take comfort that you as a doula are in the room.

Question: Do you understand how to make a space sacred for the laboring mother? Research more "sacred space for birth". What did you find?

As part of being a Comfort in Birth™ doula – the atmosphere of birth and sacredness of this time is important.

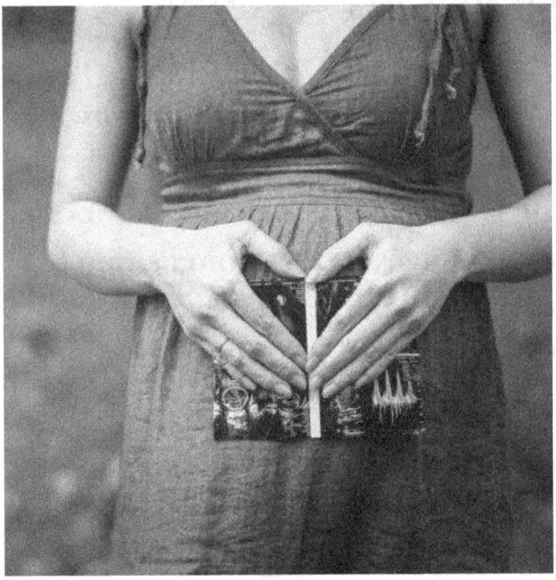

Sacredness of birth – and preparing for it are important[liii].

Trusting Relationships precursor to Birth plan or vision:

Trusting a doctor for your pregnancy care (or client's care) is sometimes risky. Does the doctor have the best interest in mind for a mother? Does a mother feel that this doctor is actually helping her pregnancy progress well? I find a lot of mothers trust the doctor without question. However, I question policies and procedures where the hospital will not allow a woman to go past 40-week due date without being induced. So, a mother may want to consider what the policies are at the hospital she plans to attend as well as her doctor's policies. Does he have a high rate of c-sections? Does the hospital allow VBAC births?

Explore More Find out what your local hospital allows concerning VBAC and inductions.

Pre-labor Signs: What can make a mom think – is this time for me to get more prepared?

1. Leaking – if mom might be leaking amniotic fluids without labor pains – this is a sign of pre-labor. She may want to talk to her provider if she thinks this is more gushing or real "water breaking".
2. Bloody show – this is usually mucous coming from the vagina that looks like a light period with mucus blood. So, this is natural – the mom can talk to her provider if she has questions.
3. Braxton-hicks contractions – those fake contractions that do not progress at all.

Positive signs of labor:

1. **Progressing contractions** – usually the rule of thumb is 4-1-1 or 5-1-1 – so basically every five minutes the mother will have a contraction that lasts around a minute long. This is also a good time to head to the hospital if you are helping a mom and she does not know when to go – go by this counting.

2. **Spontaneous rupture of the membranes** – the mother feels gushing coming out of her vagina – she is now starting real labor most likely. Have her call her provider immediately if she suspects water breaking!

3. **She is having contractions** and she is having trouble **concentrating** – then that is a good sign and that she also needs to get going to hospital right away. This means labor is progressing fast and she may even be in transition if she is not talking or having hard time talking during contractions.

Using your B.R.A.I.N.

Now using the acronym of BRAIN for the mother during labor:

B = Benefits – what are the benefits of the procedure?

R = Risks – what are the risks of the procedure?

A = Analysis – what is going on?

I = Intuition – what is the mother's intuition saying to her?

N = Nothing – what if the mother does not do anything right now? Or give her more time to see how labor progresses.

Sometimes labor takes longer to progress than expected. The doctors like to have a mom in and out of a birth within 24 hours or 12 hours or less. However, a real labor can last longer than that. Ask the doctor if mom can have more time to be left alone as long as baby is not in distress or showing any signs of trouble.

Sometimes the doctors' cause the distress by doing an epidural or other procedure.

Anyway, whatever the patient decides – they should have informed consent, know what the patient bill of rights are, etc.

Now that you have this acronym above – you can analyze a case study below!

<u>Jessica Case Study:</u>

Jessica is a teen mother about to give birth. Her mother is also at the birth to sign off on anything needed for labor and delivery. The doctors' think Jessica is taking too long in labor; she's only been in labor for 12 hours. They want to hurry things along with Pitocin. Jessica's mother is not sure. Jessica wishes to have more time, but she is not sure. You are the doula – what do you do in this situation? Also, there are no signs of distress at this time from the baby. Jessica asks the doctor what the risks are of using Pitocin for labor. You find this article to give to them:

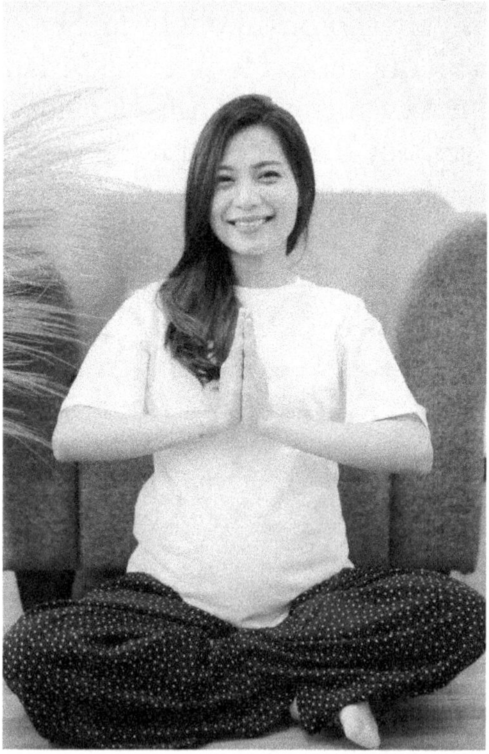

https://www.birthinjurysafety.org/birth-injuries/labor-and-delivery-complications/pitocin.html

Write out how Jessica and her mom can use their Brain better in this situation:

B-

R-

A-

I-

N-

You may finish off the scenario if so desired. ☺

Mandy Case study:
Mandy is a first-time mom. She is very nervous about birth. She saw her sister give birth and she had a lot of pain and took a while. Mandy thinks she wants an epidural and not even consider risks of epidurals or anything. She is not in labor yet, but she isn't following through with all of the consequences. Though epidurals can go fine. What can you do to help her use her Brain better?
Find her an article that show the risks of epidurals.
Then have her follow the BRAIN formula

B-
R-
A-
I-
N-

What does Mandy decide to do?

<u>**Birth Plan vs. Birth Vision or "Wishes"**</u>

Does a mother need a birth plan? And informed consent:
If a mother is going to have the baby in the hospital, yes, we think the mother should have a birth plan or birth vision. Remember to use the B.R.A.I.N. formula during an actual birth when mother needs to be informed of procedures and such. This is also called informed consent. We highly suggest having the mother explore procedures and policies for the procedures before she steps into the hospital room. If the mother is giving birth at home, she should still know what her midwife can offer or when she would have to transfer to a hospital. Look up hospital procedures that you want to know about – write down any questions for instructor.

A mother wishing to have a more informal plan may want to write out more like a birth wishes or vision statement. This can also be done in a visual way. There are several visual birth planning apps on the Internet, and some are free to find and use while others may cost a few dollars to put on your cell phone if using as an app. A formal birth plan can be done as well. **We recommend keeping it simple around 2 pages or less. Make it bulleted format on what things a mother wants or does not want done.**

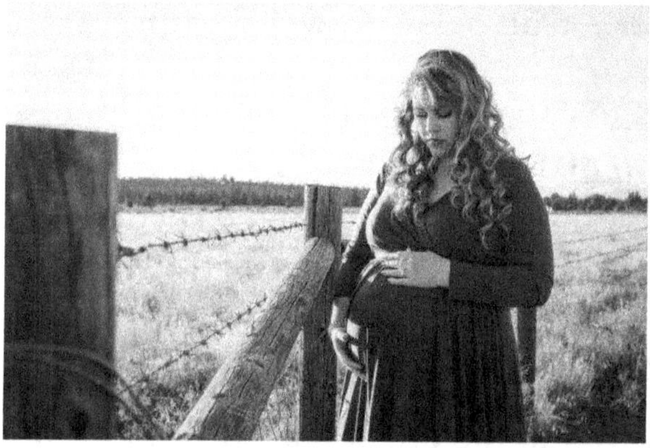

Case Study

Birth Plan or Birth Vision:

Miriam wants to have a hospital birth that feels like a home birth. She has permission to use the tealight candles that are battery operated. She is going to a "birthing suite" at the hospital as this particular hospital has one. The birthing suite has birth balls available for clients. However, this particular hospital does not allow water births. The mother may ask for a birth stool if so desired. Miriam found out she has GBS positive and will have to be tied to an IV for antibiotics when she first arrives and a few hours later if the birth is still progressing (in our scenario – we will say she has 2 IV's). Her arm will

have a heplock during the labor, so she can just get the IV in at certain times faster. Miriam is worried that the staff will suggest to her to have an epidural when she does not want one. Miriam wish list also includes skin-to-skin immediate contact with her baby if possible, cord-delay clamping or possible lotus birth (that means birthing the placenta attached to the cord), no drugs unless Miriam says a "cue word". Miriam desires her doula and boyfriend be the only ones at the birth – no students observing.

**Assignment – Write up a birth plan for Miriam and submit to instructor – read below as well for tips.

<u>Here are some tips to consider for making up Miriam's Birth Wishes/vision plan:</u>

Have a birth plan with short, bullet pointed sections that are clear and concise. (Well 2 pages should be maximum—keep it simple!)

Introduction: Who you are, who will be in the room and their role. A thank you to the providers, and an acknowledgement that you understand that birth can go in lots of directions, and you are willing to roll with how it goes. (Thank provider).

Main Goals: When I go through birth preferences, my clients pick their top three hopes for birth. Often these include a vaginal birth, or un-medicated birth. Some clients prefer to state clearly that they wish to remain with their birth team (partner and doula) at all times in this section.

Labor & Delivery: Here my clients talk about their medication preferences, whether they want to move around freely, or labor in a tub etc. This is also where clients talk about pushing and birth preferences (positions, etc.)
If there is a way to phrase something in a positive way, do it! It helps providers remember that you are friendly, kind, and wanting the best.
"Don't offer me pain medication" vs. "I will ask for pain medication if I want it." "Don't give me vaginal checks" vs. "please keep vaginal checks to a minimum." "Do not cut the cord right away" vs "We wish to Delay Cord Clamp." <u>Remember to submit to instructor the full birth plan.</u>

<u>Definitions for Doulas to look up:</u>

Terms to look up – if studying for certification – please look up terms and turn into instructor:

Apgar score
Cesarean
Contraction
Crowning
Colostrum
Complete Breech
Dilation
Effacement
Engaged
Epidural
Episiotomy
Fetal Distress
Fontanelle (Baby's head)
Forceps
Frank Breech

Induced Labor
Jaundice
Labor
Lightening
Meconium
NICU
Oxytocin
Pitocin
Placenta
Perineum
Placenta Previa
Postpartum
Pre-Term
Ruptured Membranes
Stations of baby's head
Transverse
Umbilical Cord
Vacuum Extraction

Hint on where to find terms:
https://dictionary.webmd.com/default.htm?filter=A
or https://medical-dictionary.thefreedictionary.com/
or https://americanpregnancy.org/labor-and-birth/labor-and-birth-terms-to-know/

Defining some medical procedures at birth:

- **AROM means —Artificial Rupture of the Membranes. It can be done to help speed up labor. It can hurt a lot. If a mother agrees to do this prepare her mentally by saying, —It may hurt, but you are going to concentrate on breathing and getting through this. A crochet hook like item maybe used to do this.**
- **Episiotomy is done usually while the baby is crowning to allow more room for head to slide through. This is sometimes called the —unkindest cut. Trust me a tear**

would be easier to overcome. Many women complain that —sex is never the same afterwards. So, see if alternative is available or if they perform this at all. Some places do not do this anymore.

- Pitocin: Sometimes we really do not know why labor stalls or takes longer or completely fails. Some mothers are doing fine and then all of sudden things change. Pitocin maybe given at this time to speed things up; an epidural that we thought we had rejected is given; or a C-section is given because the baby is in distress and needs to come out now! Each situation is different. Also, inductions are offered for labor not starting at certain time frames (this varies for mother or if she's having issues too) Pitocin is given in an IV. The mother will have to be tied down to a bed.
- Defining failure to progress: http://americanpregnancy.org/labor-and-birth/prolonged-labor-failure-progress/
- More info: https://evidencebasedbirth.com/friedmans-curve-and-failure-to-progress-a-leading-cause-of-unplanned-c-sections/
- See the birth challenges section for information about inductions.

Babies have their "own time" to be born. Sometimes they arrive early and sometimes "late" which is considered after 42 weeks, but some doctors will consider late even after the due date. Sometimes more incidents of meconium during birth happens after 42 weeks. The best thing to remember is that the baby will come out eventually. Is there risks to waiting for the baby to come naturally after a certain time – yes sometimes. However, weighing in are also the risks of inductions themselves. A well-monitored baby inside mommy can last as long as 43 weeks sometimes. If a mother just cannot go into labor then an induction or C-section maybe necessary.[liv]

CHAPTER 11: Introduction to Healing Arts – Part One:

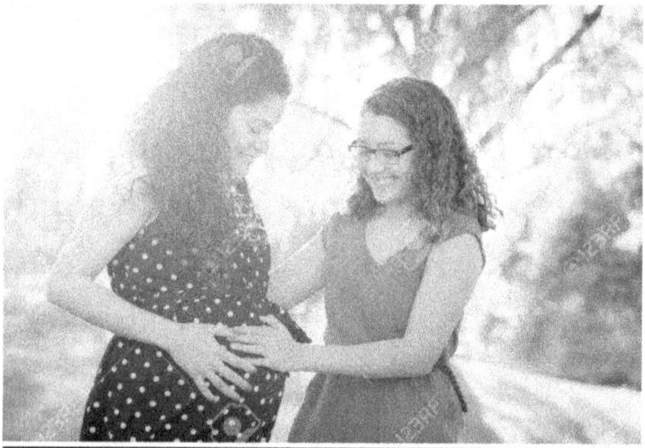

Before we get into the "all the details". Let's explain a few points here about "holistic" or "healing arts". I wanted to comment on the idea of being a "whole doula." A whole doula takes care of her clients in a holistic way. She is organized (has her forms ready for clients for instance). She is trained well (taken a doula course). She knows how to care for herself as well as her client. She answers or returns phone calls promptly. A whole doula is a bit picky about her clients. Sometimes a client is not the best fit for you as a doula – try letting go of that client then. Suggest another doula. One mistake some newbie doulas make is taking on any client that comes along. Sometimes, the mother is not the right fit, or you are not the right fit for the mother. Refer to another doula if you can. This will also get you bonus points from local doulas. They will be more willing to refer to you as well. Healing arts also means types of natural healing that may help a mother. We also want to warn you not to fall into "new agey" style. Be sure the modalities you are referring mothers too are: 1. Evidence-Based, 2. Traditional Techniques (for

example acupuncture and ancient techniques), 3. The condition the mother is seeking help from is minor not major – because she needs more doctor or midwife help if something major, 4. The healing is not rushing things (for example c-sections done before Christmas day to avoid the holiday), 5. Remember to work with other healers in your area – if you do not know homeopathy or herbs that well – then please refer a mother to an herbalist, naturopath, chiropractor, etc. You cannot do it alone and the mother is going to appreciate the referral. If you are a healer of other modalities – make sure she understands when you are using your "doula hat" vs. "herbal hat" so to speak. Be professional no matter what you offer.

Introduction to Healing Arts[lv]:

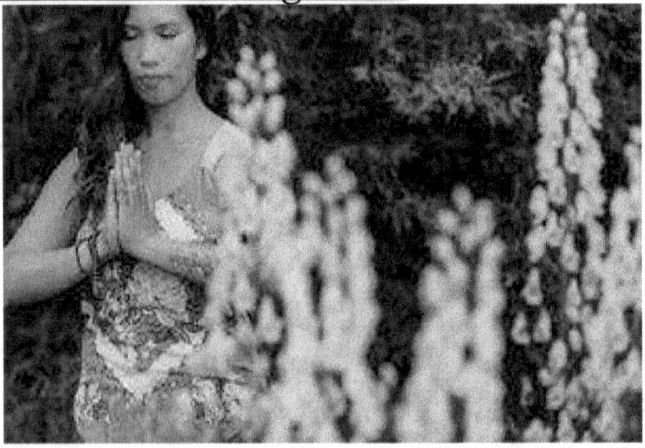

First of all, let us talk about healing and birth. After all the "H" part of comfort in birth method is healing! We go through 12 modalities or more in this chapter. We encourage you as a doula to explore learning some of these "arts" as added benefit for your clients. Mothers reading this book can learn more about these arts!

We define healing and birth as a *moment in time during a childbirth or labor experience by the mother that brings her healing from past trauma or past unfortunate birth experience.*

Here's a quote from *The Birth Conspiracy* book, "Can we heal within childbirth? This is more straightforward and includes the comforting, pain-minimizing techniques that are covered in basic doula training. These techniques can..., overcome possible traumas of childbirth, by using various healing modalities." Rivka Cymbalist.[lvi]

There are three types of healing:

1. Passive healing – we just wait and see what will happen. We may offer prayers, but in the end, it is up to God.
2. Active healing – this is when a person is ill and tries to stop the illness immediately – it is when someone like me would be taking all kinds of vitamins and such. Sometimes active healing can help; while other times it might cause more harm if you are taking too much "remedies" without any consultation from a doctor or midwife.
3. Holistic healing – this is when someone seeks to heal the "whole person" and uses precautions when it comes to medicines and does not overdue things. Holistic healing usually looks beyond just the symptoms. Holistic healing is a unique technique that not everyone can perform. Seeking the right holistic practitioner is necessary and good.

Another thing to note: Doulas are not doctors. We may offer some active or even holistic healing in the way we perform for mothers, but we do not diagnose, prescribe, or treat a mother. So, a doula is not a doctor, but she can refer mothers to other healers. Now, let's learn about some healing modalities to help mothers!

Question: **What are the 3 types of healing? How do you define healing and birth? Submit to instructor.**

1. **<u>Acupressure:</u>**

Pronounced: ak-yoo-presh-er

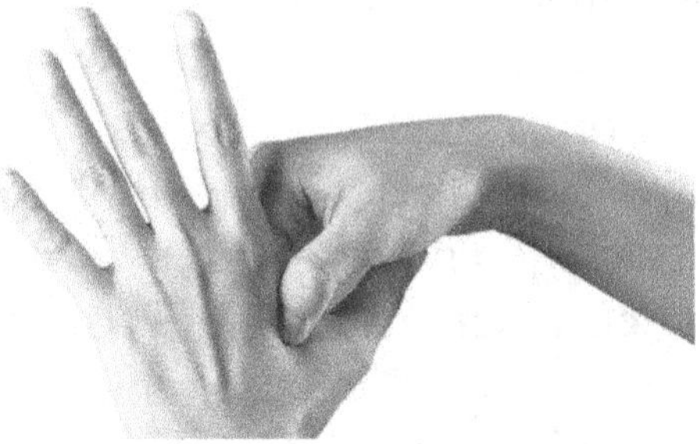

Definition: a type of massage in which finger pressure on the specific bodily sites described in acupuncture therapy is used to promote healing, alleviate fatigue, etc. They run along the same "meridian" lines as acupuncture. A meridian is a point system from Chinese medicine that is unseen and runs usually in a linear way around the human body. There are meridian charts one can find to reference to.

<u>How this can help for labor:</u> 1. Pain relief. There are a few points or areas of the body that are specific for pain relief. **2. Inducing labor**. There are a few points or areas on the body that can also help induce labor if done properly. **3. It is easy for a mother to access some points,** or a practitioner or doula can reach other points. **A mother who is familiar enough could do them a) on herself b) have a friend or relative (partner/husband) rub certain areas. A doula should avoid doing acupressure unless she is also trained in this method.**

We will mention a few spots that are popular:

Large Intestine 4 – **This is a point on your hand a spot between thumb and first finger. A mother could rub this one herself. It is useful for inducing labor and helping with pushing time. See this video for visual learners:** https://www.youtube.com/watch?v=G7wHcJiVgT4 **and locate it properly here:** https://www.youtube.com/watch?v=oy5B6D8cj1Y

Spleen 6 – **This is a spot on the mother that can help relieve a lot of maternal issues.** "It is also called the Three Yin Crossing, and it is the crossing point of the kidney, liver, and spleen meridians. This point can be found three finger widths above the inner ankle bone, along the back of the tibia."[lvii] **A mother could stimulate this point during her contractions. It also can help start up labor if mother needs that help. It is also helpful for menstrual issues and other female complaints. Here's a video for visual learners:** https://www.youtube.com/watch?v=YlVrNrcdHh4

Urinary Bladder 60 – This is another point kind of on the back area of the ankle. This point is good for circulation and provide pain relief during labor. **Video:** https://www.youtube.com/watch?v=QC0ucLYpjF8

Kidney 1 – *Mama Natural article* says: "These points pull energy downward and are typically useful during the transition phase of labor. This is also a great point for calming to help with stress and anxiety."[lviii] **This point is on the sole of the mother's foot near the depression area of the bottom of the foot.** https://www.youtube.com/watch?v=H93dqa01-wc

I apologize that we do not have access to the actual pictures. I suggest going to www.mamanatural.com to look up acupressure points on that website. https://www.mamanatural.com/how-to-do-acupressure-when-youre-in-labor/

Here is a video from YouTube about this: https://www.youtube.com/watch?v=JLz1TW8385M

There are many other points one can use. These are probably the easiest for the mother to do it herself during labor.

2. ***Reflexology[lix]:***

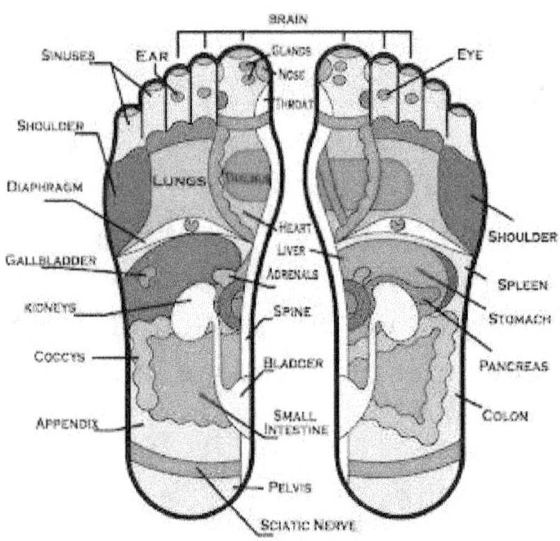

Definition: a system of massaging specific areas of the foot or sometimes the hand in order to promote healing, relieve stress, etc., in other parts of the body. See picture above. The points in the feet can be stimulated to areas of the body. Useful for helping mothers relax (before labor) or during labor and after!

The main difference between acupressure and reflexology is that the whole foot is being stimulated in reflexology – not just a particular point or area. Though the foot has several organ connections a bit like acupressure. Also, there is hand reflexology which is what we personally prefer to use during labor or birth.

You can explore more on the how and such here: Dr. Weil: https://www.drweil.com/health-wellness/balanced-living/wellness-therapies/reflexology/ School of Reflexology and more: https://reflexology-usa.org/schools/

Take time to explore more on this subject.

3. **Massage:**

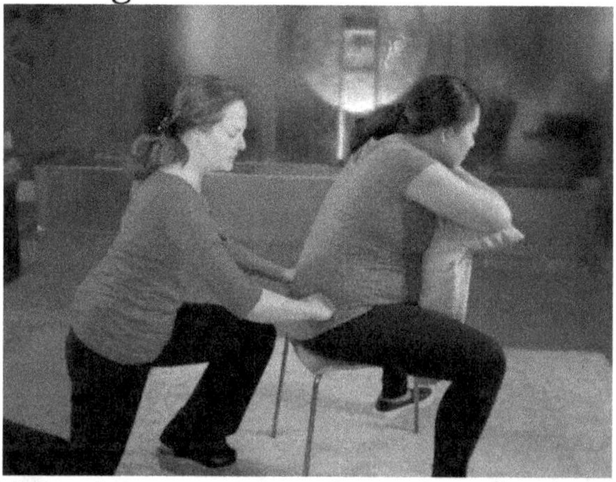

Definition: the act or art of treating the body by rubbing, kneading, patting, or the like, to stimulate circulation, increase suppleness, relieve tension, etc. This is also known as "bodywork", "havening," "light touch." As a doula we can massage a client during our work as a doula, but we are not to give massages outside our role as a doula unless we are licensed massage therapist or have a business license depending on the state you live in. ***Havening*** **is something new we found out recently about. It is basically a light touch method of stroking a mother during labor and childbirth.** It can also be done in other times. Havening starts with stroking lightly the mother's arms and shoulders. Then havening finishes at the mother's head and face. It is a unique technique. You may want "research" further to gain more insight. If you attend one of our future workshops, we will go over more of the comfort techniques in depth.

Question: Define acupressure, reflexology, and massage in your own words.

Question: How do the above techniques help a mother?

Question: Why is it best for the mother to practice acupressure and we just be the guide as a doula *Comfort in Birth practitioner?*

4. ***Homeopathy:***

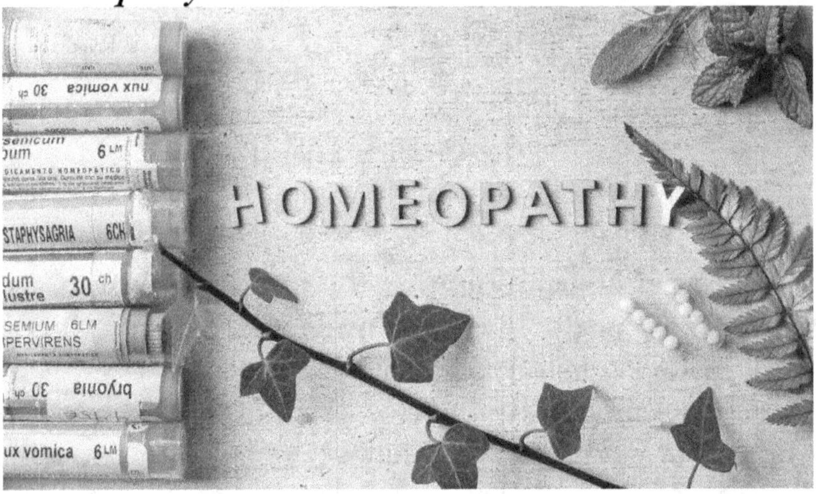

Definition: a system of medical practice that treats a disease especially by the administration of minute doses of a remedy that would in larger amounts produce in healthy persons symptoms similar to those of the disease.

Types of homeopathic medicines are somewhat herbal based, but they are the essence of the herb not the herb itself, see history info:
http://www.wholehealthnow.com/homeopathy_info/history.html
Homeopathy is harmless if your body does not respond to the remedy chosen—choose a different one.

There are some books on homeopathy and pregnancy:

1. *Homeopathy for Pregnancy, Birth, and Your Baby's First Year* by Miranda Castro (she has written other homeopathic books)

2. ***The Homeopathic Childbirth Manual:*** *A Practical Guide for Labor, Birth, and the Immediate Postpartum Period*

3. ***Homeopathic Medicine for Pregnancy & Childbirth***

We recommend reading a book before trying to pick out remedies (if a mother wants to learn) or consulting a true homeopathic practitioner. Doulas are not supposed to diagnosis, so this is a bit out realm of practice. We want to share homeopathy because it is easy to find for a mother to use and find out more on her own. One thing about homeopathy is that even if you choose a wrong remedy – there is usually little or no side effect. Usually picking the wrong remedy means you just do not get the results you were expecting. Try again! That is why we recommend finding a homeopathic or naturopathic practitioner who knows the basis of homeopathy. Now, some midwives may know this – so ask if she is trained in this or not.

5. Bach Flower Remedies:

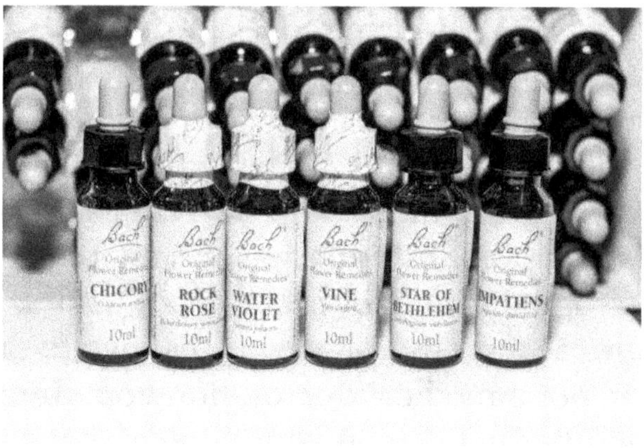

Definition: an alternative medicine consisting of a distillation from various flowers, designed to counteract negative states of mind and restore emotional balance. It is usually a tincture based and "Rescue Remedy" is the most popular to help with scary situations (kids) to helping you go to sleep (Rescue sleep), etc.

How many remedies are there?
http://www.bachflower.com/original-bach-flower-remedies

Also, look at www.backflower.com for more information. The flower remedies are great when a pregnant mother may feel scared during labor; she could put a few drops of the Rescue remedy in her water to drink. (Remember she is to ask doctor first).

6. Alaskan Essences.

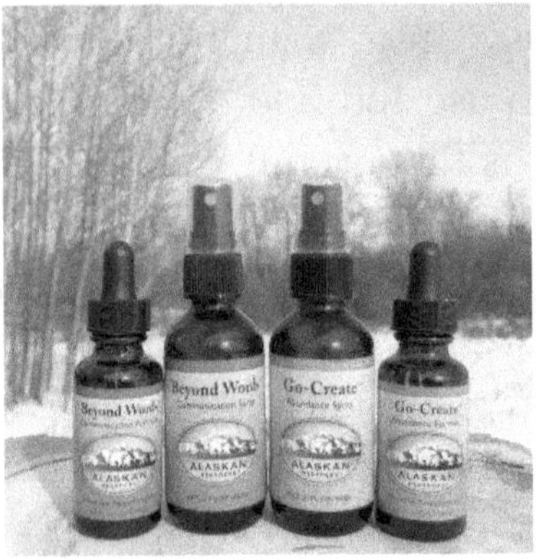

These are a bit new and/or been around for a while. They work on the same principles as Bach Flowers. www.alaskanessences.com **if you want to read more about them.**

<u>What doulas are not supposed to do:</u>

One thing we have not mentioned as much is what a doula is NOT supposed to do. I think we should take a brief break from introducing you to wonderful alternative remedies to teach a bit about this. As a doula you are here to "inform" the mother. Let her explore more and if she is super interested, guide her only! Let her make the decisions on acupressure to homeopathy and more. Now, what can a doula do? **A doula can offer the mother information and support. A doula can do light massage during labor. However, a doula should NOT ever diagnose a mother or say, "you have to take this or that." A doula is not a medical doctor, homeopathic practitioner, etc. Remember to keep on your "doula" hat so to speak when working with mothers and also know your scope of practice for your doula training. We will be adding a scope of practice statement at the end of this booklet for those who are doing the** ***<u>Comfort in Birth Method Practitioner class.</u>***

Case study time!

Here is a mini test or case study on this – we will put forth a few scenarios below – you tell us is this something a doula can do or not do?

#1 Marilla is expecting her first baby. She is 3 days past her due date and a bit impatient for labor to start. She wants you to practice acupressure on her. What would you say?

#2 Rose is a second time mother and a bit more patient. She is getting more back pain during her last trimester. She understands how to use homeopathy and already has permission from her practitioner to take arnica 30c. She just needs help opening the remedy. She will take it on her own. Can you help her open the remedy bottle?

#3 Michaela is hoping for a VBAC birth and is a bit nervous and scared. She thinks a Bach Flower remedy may ease her emotions. However, she is clueless if she should take this remedy or how much. Can you diagnosis or treat her? What can you do instead?

#4 Jodi is 39 weeks pregnant and wants to practice some massage techniques that may help her relax. Do you offer massage on her or ask a fully licensed massage therapist to do so? Why would this answer be more state specific? Look up the massage laws in your state.

#5 Nancy is in labor and just starting labor – very early stage. She is feeling nervous. She has Rescue Remedy handy and homeopathy for backaches; her doctor is out of town.

Would you be able to help her with a recommendation? (Note: Arnica is well known homeopathy for muscular pain or bruising). Find a homeopathic practitioner you could refer her too as well. (If you have one in your area).

Turn in answers to instructor if taking for full credit course. You may wish to use separate paper or email to instructor.

More Healing Arts Information:

#7 Clay and #8 Castor oil for healing. First of all, bentonite clay can be used during labor to help the mother. In one article I read, the mother can take a bit of it under her tongue during labor to help with delivery (but we don't recommend internal use). Some cultures believe taking clay will help hasten the delivery of the baby.

"Another reason given for taking the clay, "Easing labor pains, accelerating delivery, and rejuvenating the strength of the weary mother, are common cultural reasons for the use of clay for a healthy pregnancy. Clay is believed to solve nipple soreness and facilitates the secretion of milk. Also, living clay is believed to help a woman to recover from pregnancy stretch marks."[lx]

The clay can also be used on the mother's belly to help with easing labor pains. The clay also can be used on the mother's legs to help with swelling issues.

Note: There may be some side effects – so if a mother has high blood pressure – this is not recommended to take internally. We highly suggest only a mother using the clay externally. If a mother wishes to ingest, she should consult her doctor or midwife first.

Castor oil has been used for a very long time to help with inducing labor. Now, this remedy can be taken internally, but the dosage should be suggested by a doctor or midwife. Both

above remedies should be advised by the doctor or midwife, not the doula. However, you can inform the mother of these "therapies" and ask her to find out more on her own.

Question: Look up evidence for using castor oil for inducing labor. What did you find? (Name one thing you learned). Have you ever heard of using clay for any birth practices?

#9 Chiropractic for mother's healing.

Chiropractors have been part of my personal life for a long time. If you have ever been in a car accident, run to the nearest chiropractor to be evaluated. However, I find that not every chiropractor is alike. I highly recommend avoiding activator chiropractors. The activator is just a tool, and it does not work for deep tissue or other issues that mother may need help with. Also, a good chiropractor will know about alternate healing, recommend

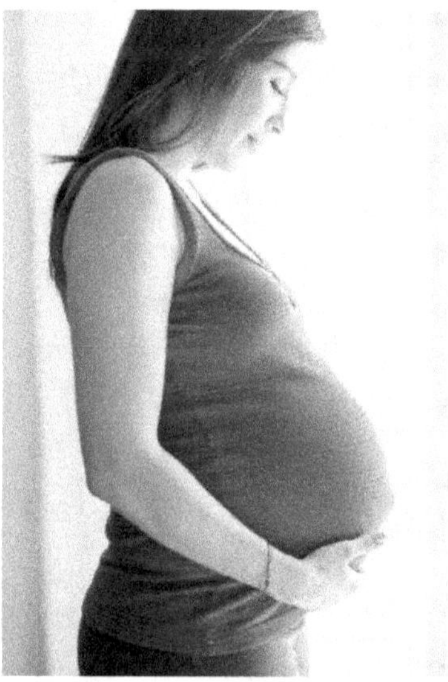

exercises to do, recommend you do physical therapy or massage, and basically be interested in the "holistic" mother and "wholistic" doula. There is a technique called Webster technique that is unique for pregnant mothers. I do not think I ever went to one like that during pregnancy; however, if a chiropractor knows "muscle testing" then this is another thing that can be helpful. Anyway, I just want mothers and doulas to know that chiropractic care varies per doctor, and you do not have to follow my recommends. This recommends not take place of a medical doctor or midwife.

#10 Water Birth!! Or Hydrotherapy! (B for buoyancy!)

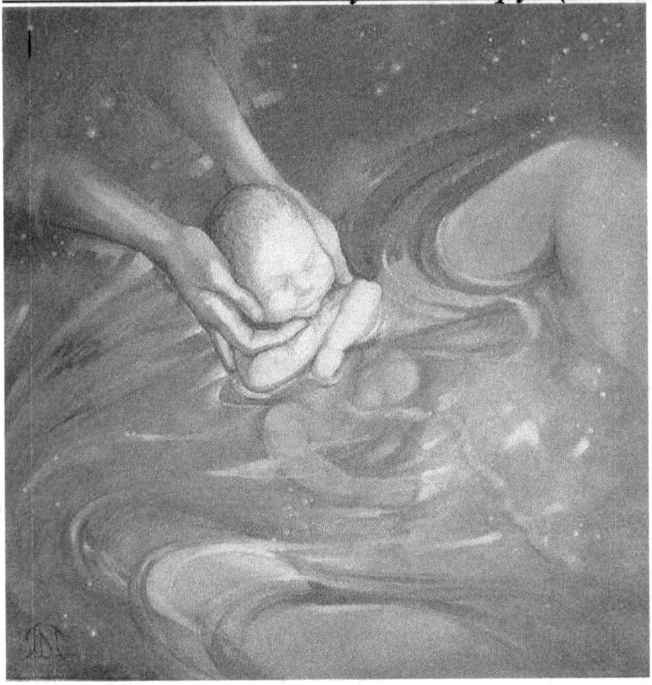

Not all births will be in the water, but a mother can use hydrotherapy (water therapy) for her delivery like taking a shower, getting in water part of the time, etc.

There are many benefits of water birth or using water during labor.

1. **It is instant pain relief for most mothers. Water with the right temperature can relieve the pain of labor.**

2. Water can help speed up labor as the mother is relaxed more in a water birth. She releases more oxytocin which stimulates the laboring time.
3. It is easier to push stage in the water. So, if a mother can push baby out in water – we recommend it – have midwife on hand to help catch baby (or let dad do the catching) and lift baby as soon as possible out of the water.
4. There's lot of evidenced based articles published that support water birth. Now, it should be done for low-risk mothers. If there's any possible high risk, then mother should follow doctor's instructions.

Question: Have you ever had a waterbirth? Research water birth and evidence for water birth. Write down 3 things you learned and quote one article you found. Are there any negatives about having a water birth?

Extra Credit Question: Have you ever heard of chiropractic care? Research to find one chiropractor in your area for your resource list for mothers.

#11 Healing Arts: Optimal Fetal Positioning

In order to gain the best birth possible, a Comfort in Birth© Doula with our methods in hand need to understand optimal fetal positioning. Spinning babies covers more on their website. We are not able to cover all of this in our manual here. We will briefly cover some of the optimal fetal positioning "language" and hopefully if a mother is reading this, it will help you as a pregnant mom understand this a bit better.

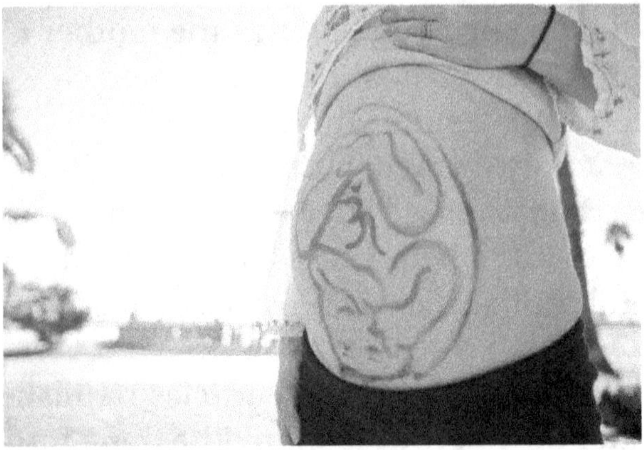

Assignment: Look up on YouTube "Belly Mapping" and practice doing this on a balloon or a real mother!

Some optimal fetal positioning terms.

This refers usually to the baby's head and position in the mother's pelvis:

Occiput – This refers to the back of baby's head, or the nape of baby's neck.

Transverse – Sideways, or laying horizontally across.

Left – The baby's occiput (back of their head) is facing left.

Right – The baby's occiput (back of their head) is facing right.

Anterior – The front of the mother.

Posterior – The back of the mother.

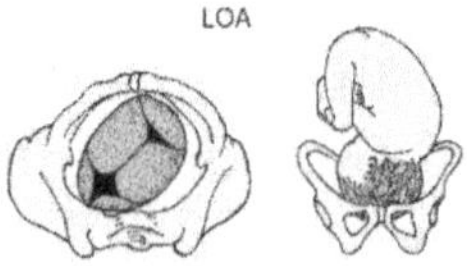

LOA: (Left Occiput Anterior) is when a baby is head-down, with the back of his head facing mama's left side and looking inward toward mother's spine.

ROA: (Right Occiput Anterior) baby's head is down, her back is facing mama's right side, and she is looking inward toward mother's spine.

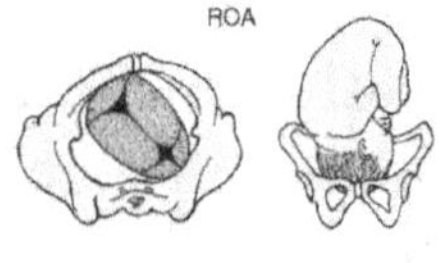

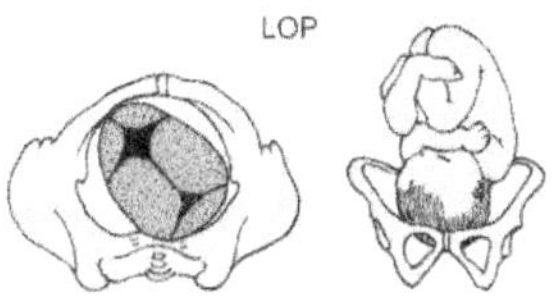

LOP: (Left Occiput Posterior) baby is head-down, the back of his neck is facing mama's left side, and his spine is up against mother's spine. In this fetal position, the back of baby's head to line up with mother's spine. (Not a very pleasant position – causes back labor).

ROP: (Right Occiput Posterior) baby's head is down, the back of her neck is facing the right side, and her spine is up against mother's spine. Again, another not so great position – can also cause back labor.

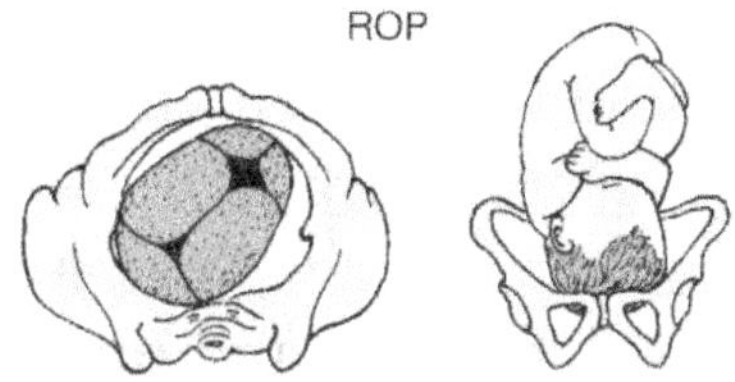

There are other positions possible, but we will stop here with these.

***Explore More: Look up some of the terms above on the www.spinningbabies.com website and that way you can "visualize" it in your head better. Please confirm with instructor that you did this. Extra credit: Work with a mother to do a belly map. Send the belly map exercise to instructor. Watch this video if you need more help: https://www.youtube.com/watch?v=uZJ9d_U3onc

<u>Time to Explore "Eye and Touch"</u>

Try this one exercise with a mother (if going in person to birth). It is called eye contact exercise. You will enter the room; if a nurse is there – you will whisper who you are to the nurse only. The mother you will approach and use eye contact only. Then you will lightly touch her hand whispering – "May I have permission to touch you and give you light hand massage (or light touch massage)." The mother will most

likely say "yes." If she says, "No." Then wait for her key to continue touching.

(Extra credit if you can do this one and share with instructor).

#12 Healing Arts Havening:

Self-havening and comfort touch for doulas:

Exploring websites about havening or self-havening – we found this information.

Definition: "The Havening Techniques are a healing modality that is designed to help individuals overcome problems that are the consequence of traumatic encoding. The Havening Techniques belong to a larger group of methods called psychosensory therapies, which use sensory input to alter thought, mood, and behavior."[lxi]

This is something new we came across when writing this booklet. So, "self-havening" is a type of touch technique for mothers that they can either do "on themselves" thus the name "self-havening" or a doula can use touch techniques that help the mother become more comfortable in birth. Since these techniques are NOT our unique ideas – we aim to link you to where you can find out more information. We like the idea because it uses "touch" as one of the senses to help mothers through labor.

Yiska Obadia is the founder of "Havening Touch". Please explore her website and videos. Her main website is http://yiskaobadia.com – We want you to go to the free videos page: https://www.yiskaobadia.com/videos Watch all the videos on the page. See below for assignment!

Here's a couple of resources for birth workers:

https://www.havenedbirther.com/

https://haveningvancouver.com/shop/

Exercise for this section: Explore the websites above –

1. Define in your own words what "havening" means to you.
2. Watch a video from Yiska's havening website and review it for a grade.

<u>Quiz over healing arts section #1:</u>

1. Acupressure is a system of putting pressure on points throughout the body. True or False.
2. Massage can help a) relax the mother, b) be used by doulas during doula work, c) all of above.
3. Reflexology can help stimulate areas throughout the body. True or False.
4. Chiropractic care can help relieve mother's back pain. True or False.
5. Bach Flower or Alaskan Essences help with what? A) Help keep a mother perpetually happy, B) Help with any emotions.
6. The use of clay can be taken internally. True or False.
7. Homeopathy is a system of a) like cures opposite, b) like cures like, c) like cures nothing.
8. LOA means… a) left occupying area b) left occipital anterior, c) none of above.
9. Havening is a system of light touch massage. True or False.
10. B is for what? (short answer)

Chapter 12: Healing Arts Part 2: Rebozo Techniques for Laboring Mothers and Exercise for Pregnancy

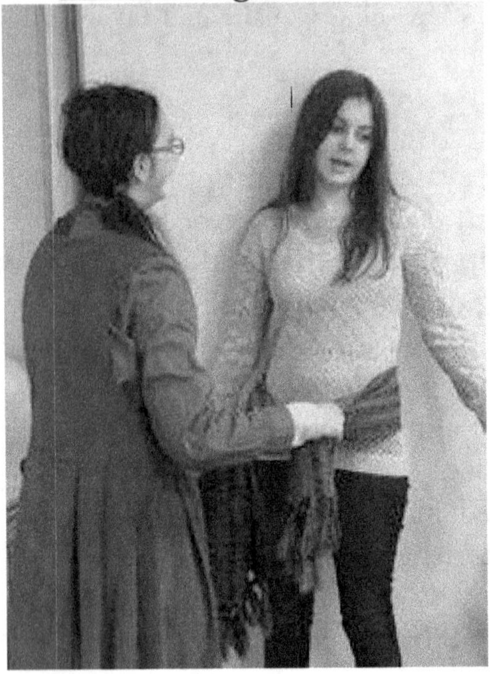

(Note: Picture is of wall sifting rebozo).

In this chapter we will be discussing our first rebozo tips and also covering birth choices. Rebozo techniques are important to offer "comfort birth" to a mother and to become a full "comfort birth" trained doula. What is a rebozo? A rebozo is a Mexican shawl (however other countries make rebozos) that is used for labor and childbirth and sometimes to carry the baby in.

The history of rebozo goes back to Mexican tradition of women wearing them as a social status and if they were married or not (different colors); these women also hid guns in rebozos during the revolutionary wars in Mexico. The rebozo seems to be a national symbol of Mexico due to this.
More about the history of the rebozo – you may want to check out these links:

1. https://www.dailymail.co.uk/femail/article-2640556/The-incredible-story-colourful-rebozo-scarf-changed-course-Mexican-history.html
2. https://www.mexican-clothing-co.com/mexican-rebozo.html

3. https://antamashop.com/blogs/antama/rebozo
4. https://mayancopal.com/blogs/news/mexican-rebozo-history
5. http://travelsintextiles.com/made-in-mexico-the-rebozo-in-art-culture-and-fashion/

Feel free to explore more about this wonderful fabric and its history.
Write down 3 things you learned from the links and send into your instructor for grading.

The Mexican style (or similar) rebozo that you receive with our program is probably around 6-foot-long (or 2 yards). However, some rebozos can be as long as 9-12 feet long. It really depends on who you buy it from, etc. Mexican sources may take 7-8 weeks to arrive.

The rebozo width also varies from maker to make; but usually they are 18 inches wide or wider. I had a "Hip Wrap" which is also a long baby carrier and I used it for longer rebozo techniques (such as Hideaway rebozo). This hip wrap is a bit wider than normal as well.

Also, Mexican rebozos can be made out of various materials. Usually cotton is common or a combo of poly and cotton. However, some rebozos are made out of silk or "silk like" material (fake silk). My favorite rebozo seller has 4 lengths for her rebozos: 1. 78 inches. 2. 98 inches 3. 118 inches or so and 4. Is XL for like carrying a baby inside.

If you want more insight into Mexican rebozo and history please purchase my book "The Rebozo Revealed" as it is longer than this section of our manual here and we highly recommend reading it!

"Light Touch" or "Tender Sleep" Rebozo (below picture):

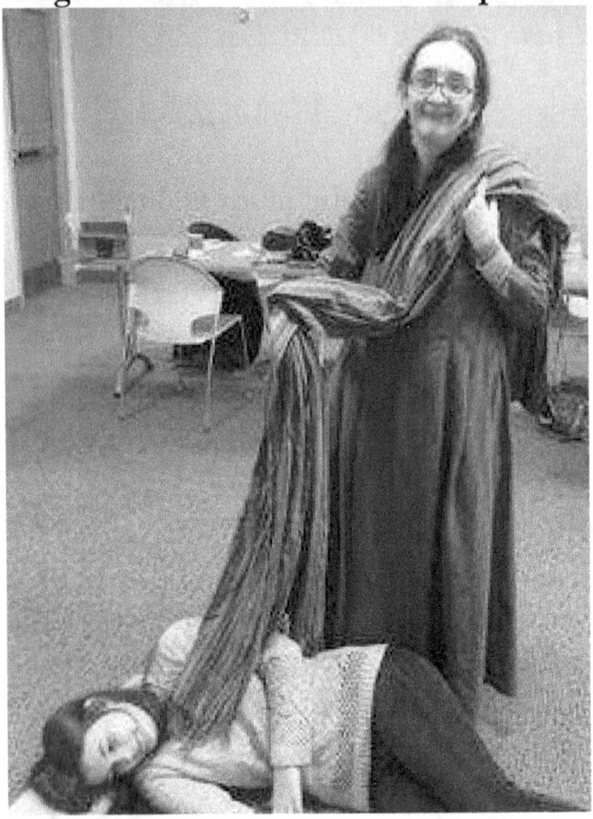

<u>How it is done:</u>

You will take your rebozo and just lightly touch your client (or friend you are working on) with the rebozo. The mother should be laying sideways if pregnant. She should also be comfortable.

Ask friend/pregnant person to take deep breaths and relax as you do this. Ask her to practice one of the breathing techniques you learned. For Example, Slow breathing.

The mother should relax in a bed or on a couch when doing this. Usually the mother is lying down; however, the mom

could be sitting up right as well if so desired. This technique can be done in early labor when mother wants to relax in bed. Precautions: Make sure mother is comfortable with her knees supported. Never have a mother lie flat on her back while pregnant.

Our second technique I call "hideaway" rebozo.

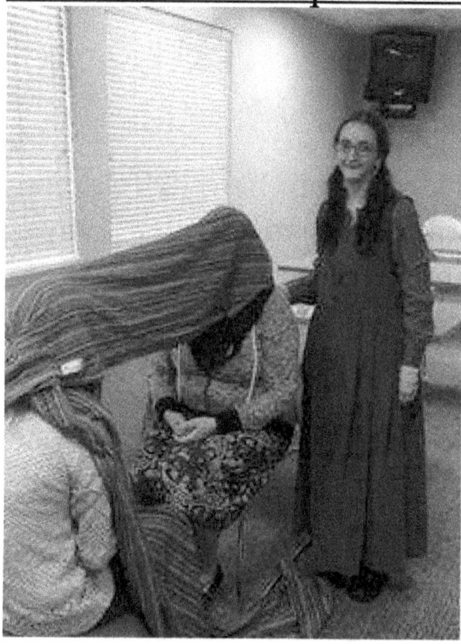

You will need 2-3 people for this technique. If you are working with a mother and her partner this is the perfect time for them to connect together under this "tent" or "hideaway" rebozo. To do this technique, have mom and her partner sit on two chairs close together. Next, cover their heads with the rebozo (making sure they can still breathe well). No giggling allowed! (😊) Have the mother and partner touch each other's arms or hands together. Ask them to practice breathing techniques together. This tent or hideaway rebozo could be done when the mother is having a hard time getting into a rhythm, this may help her focus better since all distractions are gone. If need be, put a flashlight under the "tent" area, so the couple can still focus and have some light if the room is dark. Note: Covid times some of these techniques may need to be changed up a bit.
Precautions: This one maybe hard to perform at a hospital because of the need for extra chairs.

Next technique – Get comfortable on a birth ball.

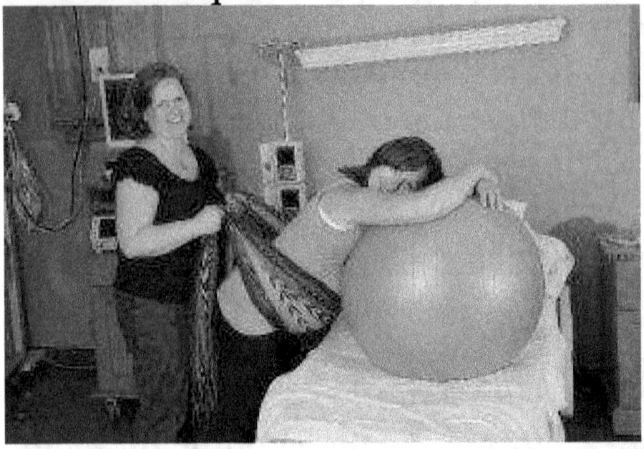

Use the rebozo to sift mother's back or just to help her sit on the birth ball for a short time. A birth ball is an excellent way to open the mother's pelvis and get her baby opening up down the "canal" to birth. This is a good optimal position. So, if mom is having some trouble with positioning, we highly recommend get her on the birth ball. This is also good practice before birth to open mother up. She could sit on a birth ball daily.

Birth ball can be done in various positions, so you can basically think about regular birth positions of sitting and leaning for instance and just add it to a birth ball routine. Mother may want to clear with her doctor or midwife if she has any special needs or high risks before working with the birth ball. In fact, none of this is to take the place of medical directives.

Many hospitals also provide birth balls, but as a doula it is always great to have one on hand. Remember to get proper sizing for mothers. (Take our Royal Rebozoway Level B for more information on birth ball www.rebozo.weebly.com)

Sifting hands and knees:

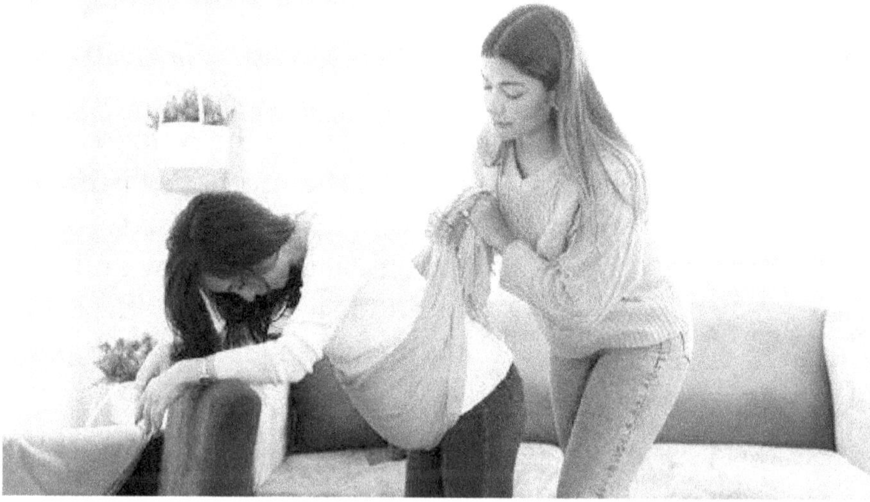

This above picture shows one way of sifting. This is probably the most common way to do sifting is with the mother on her hands and knees or leaning against something. In this picture the mother is leaning on a chair – but she could easily lean on a birth ball as well. This is a great technique to use if the baby is not in the right position (for instance posterior baby instead of anterior). Here's another picture of hands and knees:

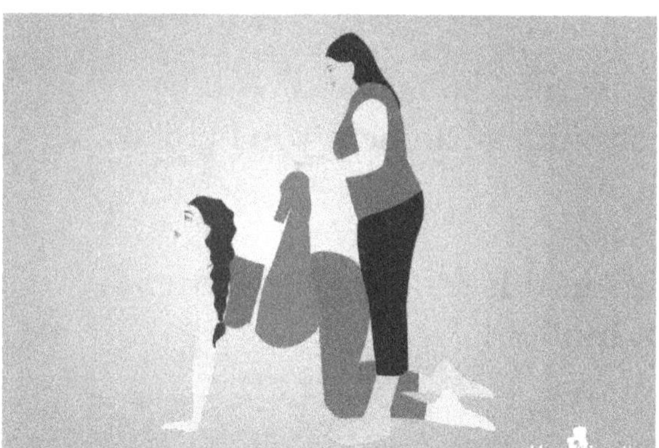

Precautions: Do not use this technique if the mother has placenta previa.

How to do this technique: Make sure you GENTLY shake or jiggle belly lightly. Also ask a midwife or doctor location of baby before doing!

Next Technique rebozo hip squeeze.

How to do the hip squeeze: *Usually this is done with your hands and your hands can get tired very easily.*

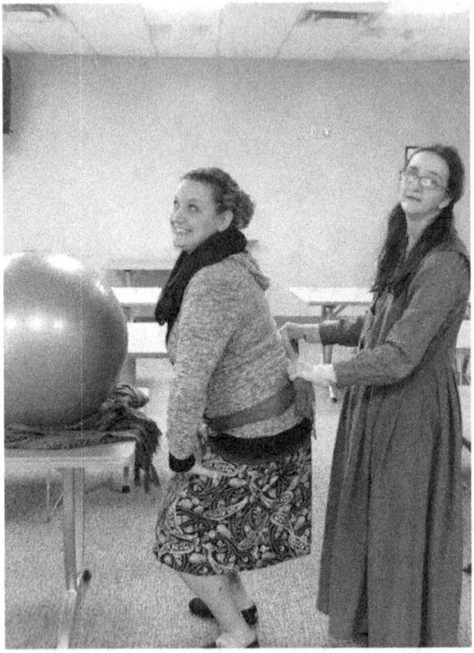

So, wrapping the rebozo around the mother's "bum" makes this technique so much easier to follow and try out! Practice wrapping the mother and squeezing with the rebozo!

Rebozo hip squeeze is great for mother's back labor or pain in that area. If she is having problems before birth, then it is time to consider some alternative healing.

You can also have the mother sit upright in a chair and you can try sifting method in a chair. This is great if mother's back is hurting during labor, and she needs a little extra relief. Try it out with a friend.

Discuss the techniques you learned so far:

How do you think these techniques can help you help a mother?

Do you have a favorite one?

Practice all of the techniques in this section with a friend, family member or pregnant mother!

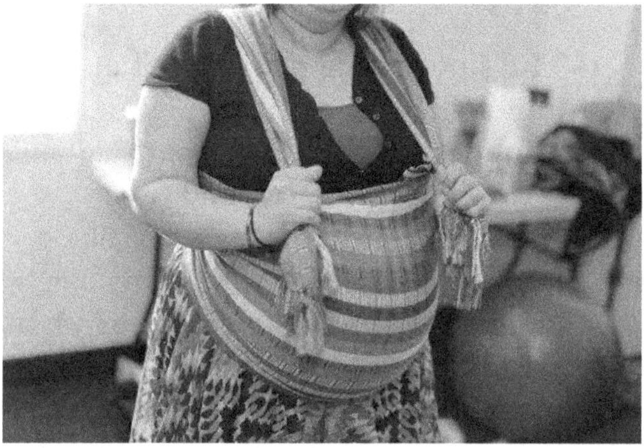

Belly Lift:

One more method – is called "belly lift" rebozo. The mother's belly is wrapped (see picture) and the rebozo is tied in the back. The belly lift wrap can be helpful if the mother is experiencing back pain during labor or in preparation before labor. Pros: This method really helps relieve back pain and can be used during pregnancy as well as labor. Cons: A mother may tire of holding this together herself – but you could use an extra long rebozo and tie it together for instance. Might be best for short time frames if mother is going to do method by herself.
How to wrap this – make sure you wrap it with an "X" across mother's back and make sure you secure the rebozo well under her belly for best support. Need more information? Look up "belly lifting" online or check out my book "The Rebozo Revealed." Thank you.

Next page for next technique…

Slow Dance Rebozo:

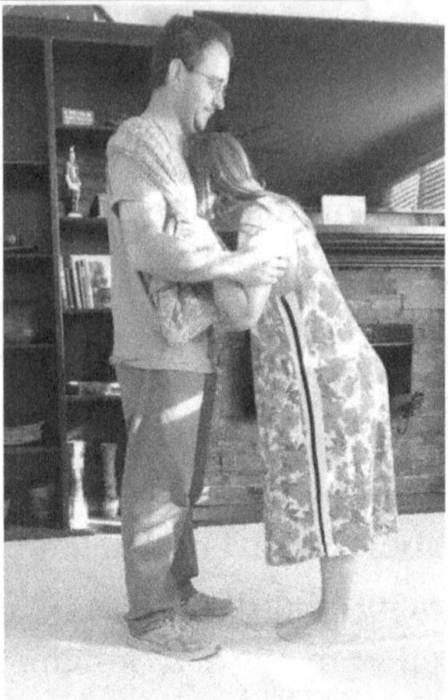

The slow dance rebozo is like dancing in pregnancy or labor. The mother can lean on her partner during a contraction and then continue a light dance when she's not having contractions. This can be great for early or mid-labor when things are not too hard for mother to stand up.

I wrote a longer book called "The Rebozo Revealed" and you can find that online at any bookstore.

Please fill out the form below for some of the rebozo skills – you need to choose at least 4 rebozo skills to complete. This is an example:

Rebozo Skill	Stars	Commentary
Light Touch	5	Sara fell asleep
Hideaway	5	We enjoyed and giggled too.
Hip Squeeze	4	Felt great – said Sara
Sifting Rebozo or w/birth ball	4	Sara liked this as well.
Slow dance	3	Sara didn't like as much

There are also rebozo bone closing or sealing for postpartum time which I cover in *[The Rebozo Revealed book.](#)* A rebozo summary picture see below[lxii].

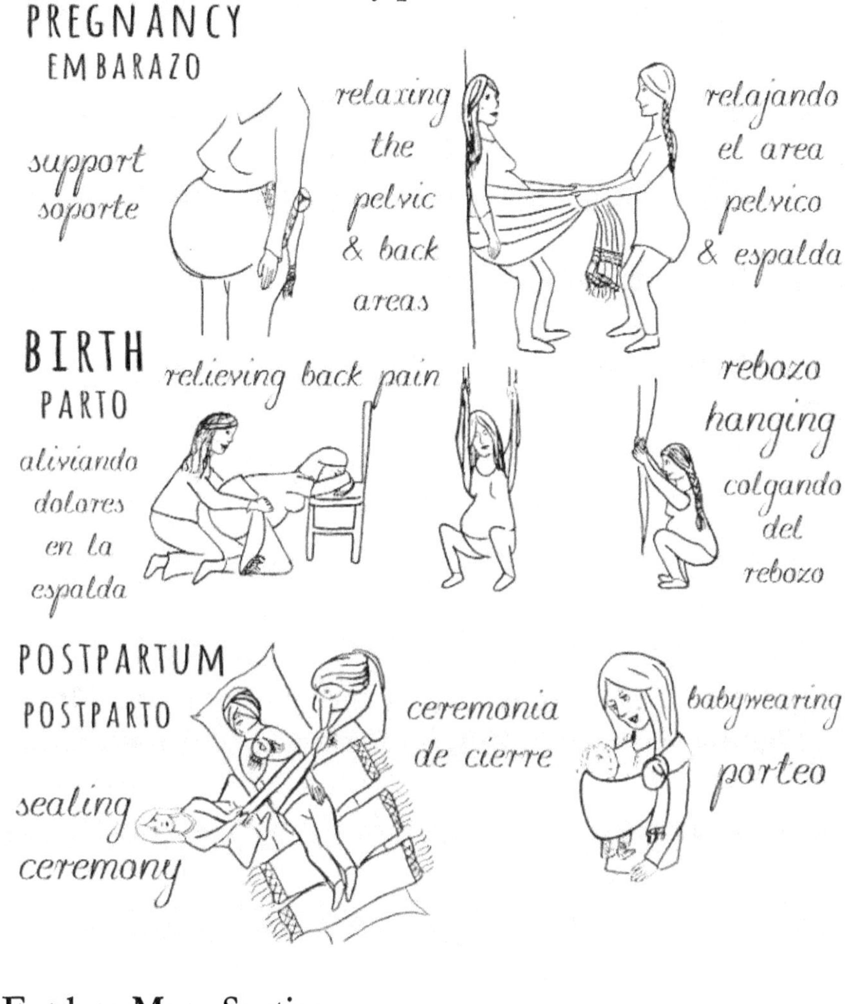

Explore More Section:

We mentioned slow breathing as a relaxation technique. We will give you some videos to look over on next slide about breathing. Different styles of breathing techniques sometimes help different stages of labor; but remember the technique does not matter as much as how the mother is coping. If she is coping well, there is no need to change her breathing patterns. If mom is not coping well, then you may ask her to try out a new breathing pattern to see if that helps!

Breathing Techniques:

Here are some video links to breathing exercises. If any links are not working, please find similar style videos on YouTube for practice!

Positive Birth company:
https://www.youtube.com/watch?v=skCJaoFSSOg
Hypno-Birthing two experts on breathing:
https://www.youtube.com/watch?v=NFucr46N308
J Breathing technique:
https://www.youtube.com/watch?v=AfGwy6Hu9-g
The Three R's and Slow Breathing by Penny Simkin:
https://www.youtube.com/watch?v=Mo4VmgpHmxs&list=PLD8uV4DMCVyHyA8QeastM0PmDSp6pMFnf

Please practice breathing exercises with a pregnant mother or a friend. Tell us how she felt before starting and then after she finished. If she felt no results – try a different technique or have her try for one week and get back to you! **Turn in results to instructor at** comfortinbirth@gmail.com

Exercise for Pregnancy – Brief overview:

The first trimester of pregnancy you may not feel like exercising that much, that is fine – do light exercise at least during this first section of pregnancy.

Second trimester – a mother should be feeling more like exercising at this time. A good routine would be to

take a walk every day and get used to movement. Some mothers like stretching exercises or Pilates. Some mothers will want to do swimming during the summer for instance. Work with whatever type of exercise you like to do.

Third trimester – a mother may slow down a little bit, but she should continue to exercise during the last trimester as this will help move the baby down the canal better.

Types of Christian programs:

Pietra Fitness www.pietrafitness.com

Soul Core (Catholic based) www.soulcore.com

T-Tapp – look it up on YouTube or "Teresa Tapp".

There's also "Holy Yoga" supposed to be more Biblically based.

Walking or riding a bike can also be great exercise for pregnancy.

Light weights can be used if so desired. Swimming can be done in summer if you like to swim.

Exercise precautions: Only exercise till you get tired – do not overdo it. Do something everyday as a habit. Always ask a doctor or midwife before starting an exercise program. Drink lots of fluids and stay hydrated. You may eat protein shakes or drinks before or after exercise. Ask a holistic nutritional coach on when the timing of shake should be done – the coach will need to know how much protein you intake and when you are eating.

Remember that nutrition and exercise go hand and hand. Make sure you are eating enough too.

Doula students' discussion: Write down one thing you learned from looking up various exercises above. What type of exercise appeals to you the best?

Chapter 13: Healing Arts Part 3: Herbs and Aromatherapy and More

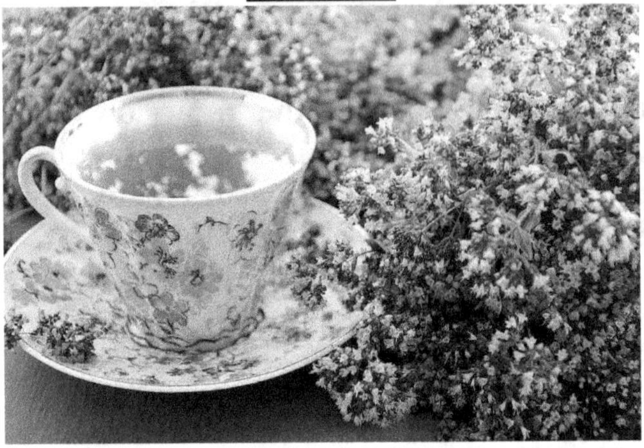

To begin with this section we will talk a little bit about "your own senses" as a type of "healing arts" or "diagnosis" tool. Though we don't diagnosis diseases – we can still use our senses to know when a mother is in trouble or not.

Our five senses are: sight, smell, hearing, taste, and feeling(touch) plus intuition!

Sight – What do we see when we first come in contact with the laboring mother? Does she look well rested or frantic? Most likely the later we will encounter. Encourage your client to rest as much as possible in between contractions for instance. If you meet with your client before labor, try to notice her surroundings and how she looks. Make a mental note of your observations and write them down later (or write them down as you talk to her).

Seeing blood – this is common for going to most births. Are you personally squeamish when you see blood? How will that affect helping mothers as a doula? Can you get over this concept?

Hearing – What do you hear in her voice? Do you hear that she seems relaxed or frantic? Maybe she sounds scared? Make sure you reassure her if she sounds like she is scared, etc. Get her to relax. Try letting go of fears exercise.

Smell – I know this one sounds a bit weird to put in here, but if a mother asks if her water has broken you can ask her what she smells! If it smells kind of earthy and something like that then her water did break. Also, if you are at a home birth things may smell different. Hospitals seem to just suck out all the natural smells of birth, but at home birth you may smell an earthy smell during laboring.

Taste – well you probably are not going to be eating much when helping a laboring mother, but a mother may want to eat something or taste something. So, keep in hand some honey sticks for instance. Honey can give the mom strength and it tastes good too.

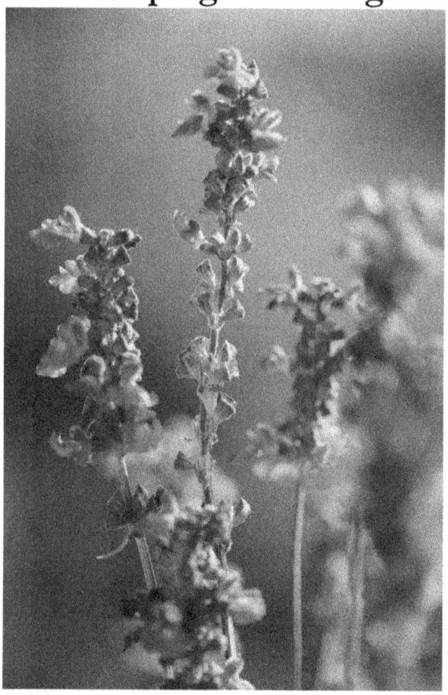

Touch/Feel: Touching is something a mother may expect during delivery of her baby. She wants to be touched and massaged. However, always ask before doing so – sometimes there are a few mothers who only want touch lightly or not much at all. Respect her space.

*Discuss the 5 senses at birth.

<u>Herbs that are safe for pregnancy.</u> We will discuss in this section a few herbs safe for pregnancy and how to use them (or best way to take) for pregnant mothers. We are not

covering the list of "bad herbs" as it is a long list. Suffice to say stick with what we discuss in this chapter as safe. These little "mini monographs" below are a short overview of these herbs.

1. Chamomile
2. Dill (safe in small amounts)
3. Echinacea (for colds)
4. Garlic
5. Ginger
6. Milk Thistle
7. Nettles (Iron)
8. Red Raspberry Leaf
9. Turmeric
10. Lavender is an herb, but we will talk about it in aroma section.
11. Spearmint is another herb that is safe for pregnancy and good to combine with red raspberry leaf for tea.
    Note: Most herbs may have indications of counteraction with drugs. Do not use herbs if taking drugs without permission from doctor. Thank you.

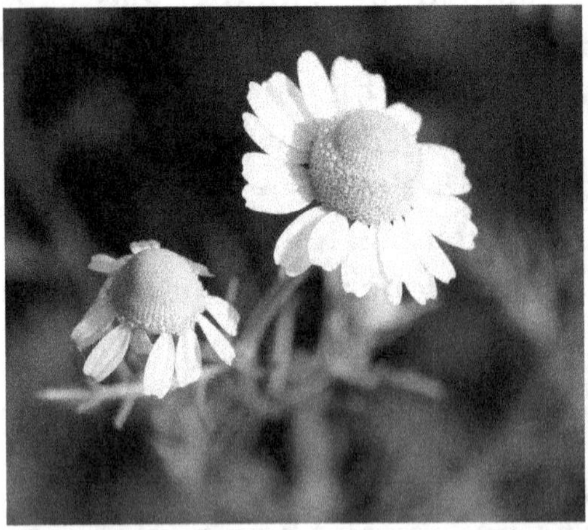

1. <u>Chamomile:</u> Use the Flowers part of this or use tea bags made up. What does it do? Chamomile is a relaxing tea and can be used for bedtime.
*Matricaria recutita is the Latin name for German Chamomile which is more commonly used for most things.
Other things chamomile can help with are muscular pain,

digestion, help with mouth sores and more. Reference https://parenting.firstcry.com/articles/drinking-chamomile-tea-during-pregnancy-is-it-safe/ *Precautions should be taken to not over consume Chamomile tea – so if pregnant a mother should limit it to one to two cups of tea a day.

2. Dill for Pregnancy: Use the leaves of the plant. Dill is popular for dill relish for instance. One article has 7 benefits of eating dill during pregnancy – includes protects from bacteria infection, dill is an antioxidant, Dill is rich in calcium and good for bone health, helps with iron levels – source of iron, and more. https://parentinghealthybabies.com/dill-pregnancy/ Side effects could include menstruation or miscarriage if overused. If a mother is worried about miscarriage wait till 2nd or 3rd trimester to use dill more. Also, always use "culinary" proportions and not overdose on dill. It could also cause skin irritation if a mother is sensitive to dill stop immediately.
3. Echinacea for Pregnancy: "In traditional herbal medicine classification, echinacea is a Category A medicine in pregnancy, indicating controlled studies in healthy pregnant women have demonstrated no foetal risk. So echinacea is one of the few herbs that can be taken during pregnancy without any worry." https://www.bioceuticals.com.au/education/article/echinacea-helps-cold-and-flu-in-pregnancy "How can echinacea help? "To support the mother's immune system during pregnancy, it may be helpful to take echinacea during any early sign of infection, exposure to infection or as a preventative during cold and flu season. Echinacea is traditionally used in western herbal medicine to help relieve the symptoms associated with the common cold, when taken at the first sign of infection." *On the other hand a mother should NOT eat goldenseal during pregnancy.*

4. Garlic for Pregnancy: If a mother wants to eat garlic during pregnancy, she should limit it to 2 to 4 garlic cloves a day. (That seems a lot to me!) A mother may want to add garlic to foods she cooks. Benefits of garlic: Can lower the risk of pre-eclampsia, boost or improve birth weight of the baby, help with cholesterol and heart issues, fight colds and infections, help with yeast infections, hair loss and more! (Article reference: https://www.momjunction.com/articles/garlic-while-you-are-pregnant_00366811/ What about side effects? Garlic can increase risk of bleeding more via C-section, if a mother is taking garlic supplements it may lower blood sugar levels if a mother is on insulin, garlic can increase digestive distress if taking a lot of it (gas, bloating, etc.) (Reference same article as above). If a mother is planning to have an elective c-section, then she may want to stop taking garlic a week or two before planned surgery for instance.

5. Ginger for Pregnancy: How to eat it: there are some ginger candies you can buy at the store or online to help with nausea, etc. You can always eat ginger root as well – use only small amounts up to one gram of ginger a day divided up into two-four doses. "Ginger Ale: while drinking soda is not ideal in pregnancy, treating nausea trumps and ginger ale is a great way to get in some ginger. The carbonation also helps many pregnant women with nausea symptoms." Source: https://avivaromm.com/5-safe-herbs-for-a-more-comfortable-pregnancy-and-better-birth/ Ginger root is best made into tea for instance or used in cooking. The benefits of ginger include helping with symptoms of nausea during pregnancy. Ginger can also help with blood circulation, colds and coughs, blood sugar levels, digestive issues like heartburn or bloating, inflammation, and tired muscles.

Avoid ginger if a mother is diabetic and taking diabetic medicines. Avoid if history of miscarriage, clotting disorders and can cause dizziness. *If you use culinary amounts as stated above, it should be safe.* The precautions are for overdoing it or if you are on any medication as well. How to use Ginger: You can use it in a tea, mince it up and include in recipes, add it to a smoothy for a spicey flavor, etc. Resource for this section: https://www.momjunction.com/articles/unexpected-benefits-of-eating-ginger-during-pregnancy_0082719/

Video about Ginger: https://www.youtube.com/watch?v=Hv2UWhJSxKY

6. Milk Thistle: Milk thistle is usually used in seed form though there are other parts that can be used. Tincture form is best way to purchase milk thistle for internal use or milk thistle as a tea form (probably the other parts are used for teas). Benefits of Milk thistle for pregnancy include morning sickness, mood stabilizer, increase breastmilk production (for postpartum), benefits liver, supports kidneys, supports diabetes, antioxidant, etc. What are the cons for this herb? It might cause nausea; it may cause diarrhea and it might cause allergies if someone is allergic then the person should discontinue use. Source of information: https://parentinghealthybabies.com/milk-thistle-pregnancy-nursing-benefits/

7. Nettles: Stinging nettles or *Urtica dioica* is a common weed! So, some weeds are good for you. Preference for pregnancy would be a tea form – less strong and still has plenty of benefits. It also can be found in tincture form.

What are the benefits of Stinging Nettles from Wild Mother Life blog: "Nettle infusions are extremely high in calcium and magnesium. Some sources say that one quart of a nettle infusion contains 1000mg of Calcium and 300mg of Magnesium! For reference, that amount meets the daily recommendation for women for both calcium and magnesium. Nettle also contains Vitamin A, C, E, F, K, Zinc, magnesium, iron, copper, selenium, boron, bromine, chlorophyll, potassium, phosphorus, iodine, chromium, and many of the B Complex Vitamins. It also has more protein than almost any other plant. Nettle Leaf is extremely nourishing and has little to no side effects, therefore I think it's a perfect herb to drink during pregnancy! To play it safe, the general rule of thumb for consuming any herb is to wait until after the first trimester. I personally drank nettles all throughout my pregnancy and felt quite safe doing so. However, the second trimester is a great time to start drinking nettle as well! The general rule of thumb for nettles is to allow the herb to steep overnight. The ratio should be around 1-3tsp of herb per cup of hot water. Using 3tsp of herb will make a really strong brew and using less will be a little less strong. The easiest way to make it is to let it steep in a French press overnight! Best place to buy high quality nettles is from Mountain Rose Herbs." End of quote. I want to add in that Wise Woman Herbs has Nettles in tincture form as well. Source for this article: https://wildmotherlife.com/nettle-tea-pregnancy/

8. Red Raspberry Leaf: Red raspberry leaf (Rubus idaeus) for an easier labor. This herb is a mineral rich tonic, traditionally used to support a healthy pregnancy and tone the uterus to help a woman prepare for birth. Some studies have shown that it can help to expedite labor and reduce complications and interventions associated with birth. Since it doesn't have the most pleasant taste when taken as a tea by itself, (Aviva Romm) I generally recommend mixing it with some spearmint and rose hips for a delicious tea that can be taken daily, 1-2 cups throughout the second and third trimesters. The recommended dose is from 1.5 – 5 gm daily in tea. Pregnancy Tea: 2 tbsp red raspberry leaf + 2 tsp spearmint leaf + 2 tsp rose hips. Mix together and place into a reusable tea bag. Steep in 8 oz of boiling water for 20 minutes, strain and drink 1-2 cups daily. Source:

https://avivaromm.com/5-safe-herbs-for-a-more-comfortable-pregnancy-and-better-birth/

9. Turmeric: **Fresh or dried turmeric is likely to be safe when pregnant women consume it in small amounts, e.g., the amounts typically found in meals, such as curries and other dishes. Pregnant women should avoid taking medicinal quantities of turmeric. This includes capsules or supplements containing turmeric or curcumin, which is its key active ingredient. Ground turmeric used in cooking contains lower amounts of curcumin than supplements.**

   Benefits of Turmeric: Can help with excess inflammation, fetal brain development, and oral health support. How to take turmeric – try sprinkling it on your vegetables or stews, adding it to smoothies, add it to milk, etc. Only use culinary amounts for pregnancy.

   Source: https://www.medicalnewstoday.com/articles/turmeric-during-pregnancy#is-it-safe

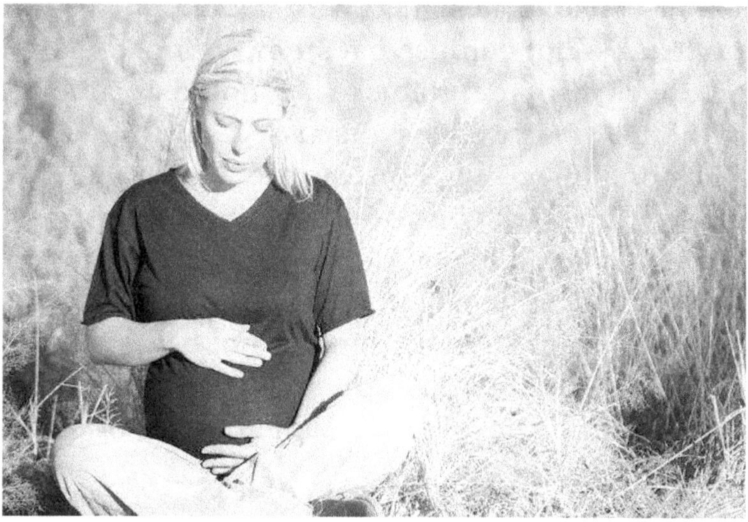

10. Lady's Mantle (Alchemilla vulgaris) Leaves[lxiii]: This is not used as much in America, but Europeans use this herb more. It is a great herb for helping with hemorrhaging during childbirth. It can also help settle an upset stomach and is useful in treating morning sickness.
11. Lemon Balm[lxiv] (Melissa officinalis): This "herbal" remedy so to speak is not commonly used for pregnancy but it is safe. It can help calm the nerves and relax the mother. It is great as tea with a touch of honey added. It can also help with a headache, mood support, and insomnia! Add Red Raspberry as a tea combo. It also helps with digestive issues.
12. Oat Straw stalk and unripe fruit: (Avena Sativa). This herb is rich in calcium and magnesium and great served as a tea for stress reduction for pregnant mothers. Also, tastes good with chamomile combined into tea. Do not confuse oat straw with oatmeal – this is completely different items! You should be able to find any of the herbs we have discussed at Mountain Rose Herbs online. www.mountainroseherbs.com
13. Slippery Elm Bark[lxv]; Another safe herb for pregnancy. This one is good for supporting colds, flus, coughs, illnesses, etc. It helps mucous membrane inflammation or irritation. It is a myth about it not being safe is because of a bad Native American practice which has to do with the sticks not the actual leaves or tea portion of the slippery elm.

Herbs to AVOID during pregnancy[lxvi]:

1. Black Cohosh and Blue cohosh – both have similar properties as a uterine stimulant and uterine relaxant.

2. Motherwort- though it can be used towards very end of pregnancy – but it is not recommended during pregnancy as it can produce uterine contractions.
3. Pennyroyal leaf and oil: This can stimulate blood flow to the uterus and pelvis area (Great for PMS) – however it is toxic and should not be used during pregnancy.
4. Shepherd's purse use cautiously. However, it can be used after the baby is born for hemorrhaging – just don't use during pregnancy. The herb should be used fresh or tinctured if doing for hemorrhaging reason.
5. Yarrow is an excellent hemostatic and can be used with Shepherd's purse for hemorrhaging – just don't take during pregnancy!

Pregnancy Tea Recipe:

3 parts red raspberry leaf, 3 parts lemon balm, 2 parts nettle, 1 part alfalfa leaf (also safe for pregnancy), 4 parts spearmint (possibly peppermint – but spearmint is better for pregnancy). A pinch of stevia.

Mix together in a bowl. Use 4 to six tablespoons of herb mixture per quart of water. Place herbs in cold water and bring to a simmer over low heat. Immediately remove from the heat. Keeping the pot covered, let mixture infuse for twenty minutes or longer and strain.[lxvii]

Case Study for Herbs A:

Adeline is pregnant and was told that she is borderline anemic. She also could use a good vitamin boost. What herb from above would help with these issues? What way would you recommend Adeline take this herb?

(With permission from doctor – we will pretend each case study mother has permission to use herbs or aromatherapy).

Case Study for Herbs B:
Beatrice is pregnant and has nausea and is also having issues sleeping. What one or two herbs would you recommend for Beatrice to try using to help this?

Case Study for Herbs C:
Cassie is pregnant and has a lot of mucus problems from a cold. She wants to know if she can make a tea out of slippery elm or not safely?

Case Study for Herbs D:
Dina has an upset stomach and also trouble sleeping at night. What two herbs would you suggest she try out? Why?

Case Study for Herbs E:
Eleanor wants to try drinking a combo tea using the following ingredients: lemon balm, red raspberry, and blue cohosh. *What ingredient should she remove?*

Submit all to comfortinbirth@gmail.com *or* *catholicdoulanews@gmail.com – thank you.*

Aromatherapy for Pregnancy

What is aromatherapy? **Definition: inhalation or bodily application (as by massage) of fragrant essential oils (as from flowers and fruits) for therapeutic purposes.**
Broadly: the use of aroma to enhance a feeling of well-being. (Source Merriam Web Dictionary).

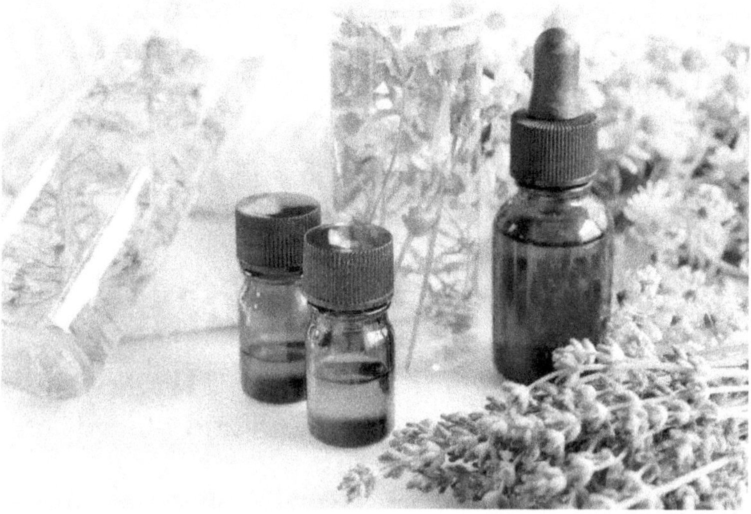

Safe for Pregnancy Essential oils and a little bit more about oils in general. If an oil is not safe or unknown for pregnancy - we will put a "star" * by it.

1. Bergamot Oil: Bergamot is one of the great essential oils for pregnancy use. This oil has many benefits including anti-fungal, anti-bacterial, and anti-viral. Bergamot is a citrus oil, giving it a very fresh scent that you will enjoy. In addition to its health benefits, it is also excellent for boosting your spirits naturally and decreasing stress. Though it is not on the list in the Aroma book I have - I think use with precaution during pregnancy -later trimester.

2. Grapefruit Essential Oil is another citrus essential oil for pregnancy that is great for beginners and has multiple benefits. Citrus oils, like grapefruit, are a great way to fight fatigue, boost your mood, and decrease stress. Place the drops of Grapefruit in your diffuser to begin filling your home with delicious scent and at the same time boost your home's mood and immunity!

3. Lavender Essential Oil: Lavender is one of the best essential oils in my opinion. This oil smells heavenly and has a list of benefits.
   Lavender is a great remedy for:
   Headaches/migraines
   Insomnia
   Nausea
   Aches/pains
   Anxiety/stress and safe for pregnancy. TIP: Try adding a few drops to a warm, wet washcloth and place it on your head for headache relief.

4. Chamomile Essential oil:
   One of the greatest benefits of Chamomile is using it as a sleep aid. Place a diffuser in your bedroom at night and diffuse while you get ready for bed. This is a great oil to help with relaxation and treating pregnancy insomnia. (Yes, safe for pregnancy).

5. Eucalyptus Oil: One of the benefits of eucalyptus oil is its ability to help relieve many cold symptoms. But is eucalyptus oil safe during pregnancy? Current data suggests that this oil can be used safely during pregnancy. Eucalyptus essential oil can be used to treat congestion, clear the sinuses, and provide pain relief.

To use eucalyptus essential oil for pregnant women, combine 1-3 drops of the oil with a carrier oil and pour into the bath. Inhaling the oil will promote relaxation while helping to clear up any respiratory problems.

6. Frankincense essential oil*** has many benefits and has been used during pregnancy to maintain and promote healthy skin. It can help treat minor blemishes, soothe dry skin, and even heal wounds. Because of its ability to maintain healthy skin, frankincense is one of the essential oils for stretch marks during pregnancy. While many women have used this oil safely, there are conflicting opinions, and you should always consult with a qualified professional before using frankincense essential oil while pregnant. ***Because of above we do NOT recommend during pregnancy but to wait till after or consult a certified aromatherapist first.

7. Rose Essential Oil Pregnancy: Another oil with a delicate floral scent, there are many benefits of rose essential oil. This oil is known to revitalize the skin, reduce stress and increase relaxation, making it a great choice for pregnant women. Mix 2-3 drops with water in a diffuser and let fill the room. Or, use topically by combining 2 drops with 1 Tbsp. of carrier oil and massage over the skin.

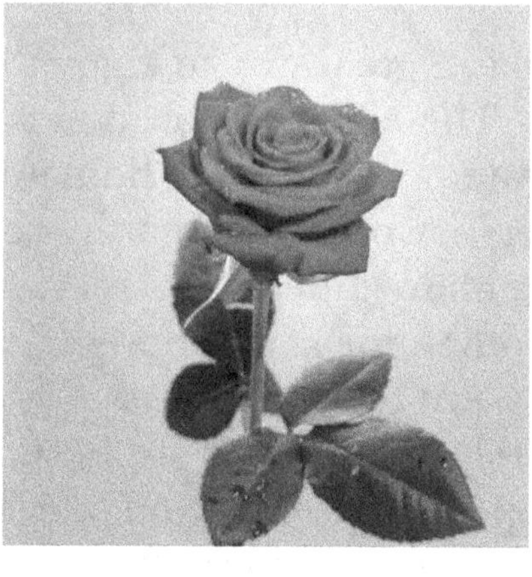

8. <u>Douglas fir essential oil</u> has a fresh, woodsy scent and is

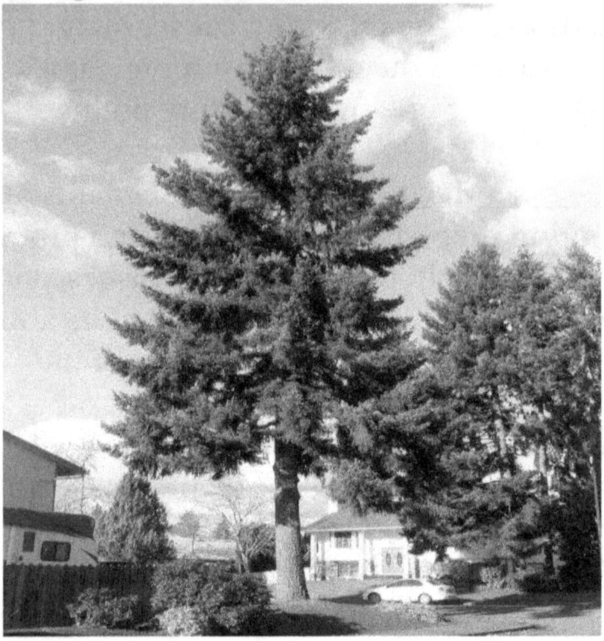

used in aromatherapy for its many benefits. The oil can help to ease anxiety and stress, improve sleep, and boost energy levels or *support mood.* It is also used to treat respiratory conditions such as bronchitis, coughs, and colds. The Douglas fir tree is native to North America and grows in the Rocky Mountain region. The oil is extracted from the needles and twigs of the tree.

   Douglas Fir Essential Oil is a great way to enjoy the benefits of aromatherapy. The oil can be used in a diffuser, added to bath water, or made into homemade products. The oil has a fresh, woody, and earthy scent that can be used to create many different recipes.
9. <u>Lemon essential oil</u> is another one safe for pregnancy and will add a nice fresh scent to any combo.
10. <u>Lavender Essential oil</u>: Helps with mood support, antioxidant, diabetes support, brain function, etc. It is basically the go to oil for almost anything. Lavender also has been known to help with burns.

Here's a video on how to make essential oils:
https://www.youtube.com/watch?v=mMr-Ux5S8vY

Essential oils NOT safe for pregnancy or breastfeeding list - from Aromatherapy & Essential Oils Handbook! List below: Aniseed, Star Anise, basil, bay laurel, birth-sweet, carrot seed, cinnamon, fennel, hyssop, jasmine, Spanish lavender, lemongrass, Melissa, myrrh, myrtle, parsley, ravinstara, sage, Spanish Sage, savin, tansy, tea tree oil (lemon variety), thuja, thyme with lemon, verbena with lemon, wintergreen, wormwood, and yarrow. So, avoid all of these during pregnancy or breastfeeding. If you are NOT planning to breastfeed - then you might be able to use after baby is born.

Safe Essential oils list:
Safe for pregnancy list (From Aromatherapy Handbook):
Benzoin, Roman chamomile - not German, Douglas fir, silver fir, geranium, ginger, grapefruit, juniper berry, lavender, lemon, mandarin, neroli, sweet orange, palmarosa, patchouli, pine, rose, rosewood, thyme, ylang ylang.
Postpartum care: Roman chamomile, clary sage, frankincense, geranium, grapefruit, lavender, patchouli, rose.

How to dilute essential oils: See this chart picture:

Carrier oil	1%	2%	3%	4%	5%
1/3 oz / 10mL / 2 tsp	2 drops	4 drops	6 drops	8 drops	10 drops
1/2 oz / 15mL / 1T	3 drops	6 drops	9 drops	12 drops	15 drops
1 oz / 30mL / 2T	6 drops	12 drops	18 drops	24 drops	30 drops
2 oz / 60mL / 1/4 c	12 drops	24 drops	36 drops	48 drops	60 drops
4 oz / 120mL / 1/2 c	24 drops	48 drops	72 drops	96 drops	120 drops
8 oz / 240mL / 1 cup	48 drops	96 drops	144 drops	192 drops	240 drops

Carrier oils can be olive oil, coconut oil, sesame oil, etc.

Morning sickness blend:
20 drops of lemon essential oil
20 drops of ginger essential oil
20 drops of spearmint essential oil
What dilution rate is above combo of oils? How much carrier oil do you need for this rate?
In a 5 ml. glass dropper bottle, combine all oils and shake to blend. You can apply topically.

You can also make an air spray or diffuse in the air or inhale it. NOT to be used internally.

Varicose Veins Essential oil recipe
4 tsp. of grapeseed or almond oil (carrier oil)
10 drops of geranium essential oil
10 drops of neroli essential oil
5 drops of cypress essential oils (If using for pregnant mother check safe list and drop an oil if need be).
Combine together in a bottle.
Can you figure out the dilution rate of the above oil combo?
Mothers may use on legs once a day.

Maria Case Study:
Maria is a pregnant mother who wants some suggestions for essential oils to use for following symptoms - remember you are not diagnosing just helping with suggestion:
She has nausea or morning sickness, She has trouble sleeping, She wants to relax more.
What 2-3 oils could you suggest? And Why?
Or you may suggest a blend for her to take.
Added question about dilution: Let's say you are making her two oil combo for pregnant mothers it should be 1% dilution – see chart and figure out how you would accomplish that – write down 5% dilution for 2 oils and 3% dilution for 1 oil and submit to instructor for grading.

Stacey Case Study:
Stacey is a pregnant mother who wants some suggestions for essential oils to use for following symptoms:
Stacey has back pain. Stacey is restless and has insomnia. She has varicose veins. She feels a lot of pressure in her pelvis. Stacey is in her third trimester. Suggest 2-3 oils she could use safely right now.
How would you dilute the 2 oils you have chosen for Stacey?

Case Study Peggy: Peggy is in labor and wants some oils to use for her labor time. What oils are safe for her to use?
She also wants one suggestion for a breastfeeding safe essential oil to use immediately after birth just in case she is anxious or needs something to help her relax.

Submit to instructor the case studies. Thank you.

Remember to consult a physician, aromatherapist (certified) or herbalist before using herbs or essential oils officially AND do your own research on anything and everything.
Doulas are to NEVER diagnose any mother.
Safety first!
Resources for aromatherapy section:
https://justsimplymom.com/the-9-best-and-safest-essential-oils-for-pregnancy-a-beginners-guide/
And: https://essentialoilexperts.com/essential-oils-for-pregnancy/

Short Quiz over herbs/aroma:

1. We first talked about five senses at birth. Does birth have a smell. True or False?
2. Which herb below "Can lower the risk of pre-eclampsia, boost or improve birth weight of the baby." A) Ginger, B) Garlic, C) Turmeric, D) Chamomile
3. Which herb below "can help with relaxation and sleep". A) Nettles, B) Chamomile, C) Milk Thistle, D) Garlic.
4. Which her below "can help with raising iron levels" and has lots of other vitamins in it? A) Dill, B) Echinacea, C) Chamomile, D) Nettles.
5. Which herb can help with liver support? A) Echinacea, B) Nettles, C) Milk Thistle, D) Garlic.
6. Douglas fir essential oil is good for what conditions? A) mood support, B) sleep, C) coughs, D) all of above, E) A and B only.
7. Rose essential oil can NOT do one thing below: A) Reduce Stress, B) help mother relax, C) help the skin, D) help with a cold.
8. Lavender essential oil can help with what? A) Brain function, B) Burns, C) Mood support, D) all of above, E) A and B only.
9. True or False: Frankincense oil is 100% safe for pregnancy.
10. True or False: Sage Essential oil is 100% safe for pregnancy.
11. True or False: Spearmint herb can be used along with Red Raspberry herb for pregnancy tea. True or False.
    Submit Quiz to instructor.
12. True or False. Caroline can take slippery elm tea safely as a pregnant mother.
13. Maria is going to drink lemon balm and black cohosh tea. That's OK for pregnancy. True or False.

Chapter 14: Healing Arts Part 4: Self-Care for the mother and unassisted birth information

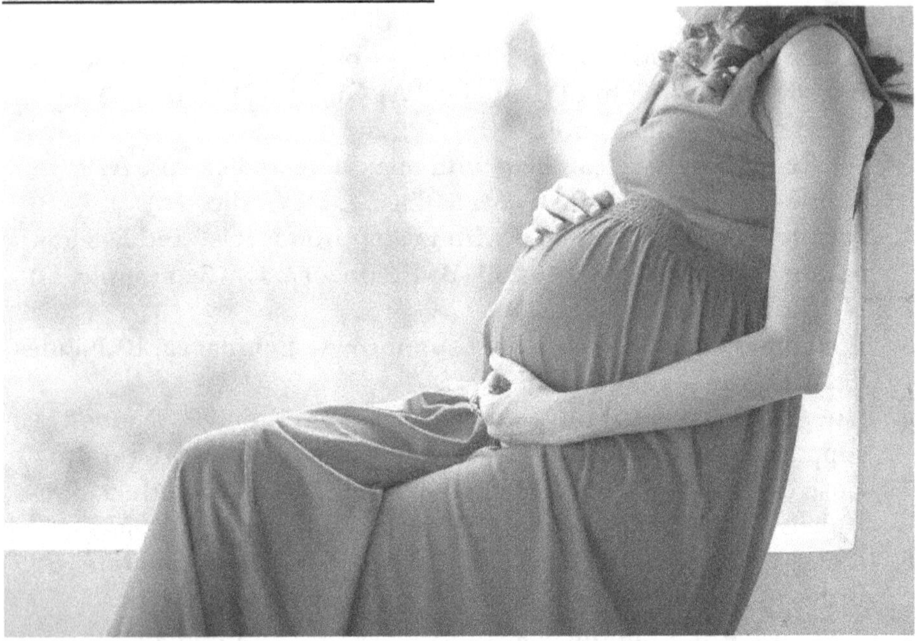

Have you thought about pregnancy and childbirth as a healing ritual? Can birth be healing? Yes, childbirth can be healing esp. if a mother has had a past trauma, etc. The reason for creating Comfort in Birth Technique is to give mothers an opportunity for healing. One way of healing is "self-care."

Ways of healing include taking care of yourself (if a mother is reading this) or as a doula we need to make sure the mother is getting "self-care" time in during her pregnancy (prenatally) is very important. If a mother takes time for herself during pregnancy this can also help, be a preventive for postpartum depression.

Let's use our Acronym of COMFORT to come up with ways to do self-care.

C = Calm, Comfort, caring: As a mother who has had a few babies, pregnancy can be worrisome and stressful sometimes. Taking time to stay calm and care for yourself is important. Create a plan to help yourself be comfortable in pregnancy. Make a fun daily routine to help you relax and be confident in your pregnancy. A simple routine could be for example: Red Raspberry Leaf tea in the morning with breakfast, go out and get sunshine by going for a walk after breakfast. Sit and read a pregnancy book, etc. If you are a pregnant mom that is working, then think of having a short break during work time to relax or read. Doula Tip: Remind moms to stay Calm – remember our other acronym – C for Christ, A for Allow, L for Love, and M for Mothering. Use the Letting go of Fears exercise as needed too.

O = Oxytocin, Oxygen, Open Air: This self-care technique is important – many mothers like having "sex" more during pregnancy esp. 2nd or third trimester. It is actually fun and won't hurt the baby at all. (However, avoid if you are leaking amniotic fluid). Next is oxygen – that means trying some breathing exercises as part of your daily routine. You can look up breathing exercises on YouTube. Open Air – well just like that – go outside like mentioned above and get some sun and Vitamin D (naturally) from the sun! Doula Tip: Remember to remind mother to go out and get some sunshine!

M = Mothering yourself, Meditation/prayer, etc. This self-care technique goes back to a more spiritual practice in away – you are taking care of mothering yourself by prayer for instance. Also, meditation is known to help calm nerves and open yourself up to opportunities. Practice whatever kind of meditation you like if Christian you may want to consider a "snapshot" of Christ's life. Meditate on a Rosary mystery if

Catholic, etc. Doula Tip: Remind mother to consider a spiritual practice during her pregnancy.

F = Feelings/Emotions – Do joyful activities: This self-care technique focuses on emotions and feelings. You may want to start a pregnancy journal for instance and write down how you feel each day. Journaling is a good way to let go of frustrations, anger, etc. Replace any frustration with Joy! Think about your baby coming soon. Write little "love letters" to your baby is one other idea! Think of a happy thought each time something sad tries to enter in. Doula Tip: Remind mothers to do pregnancy journaling.

O = Opening up to Allow yourself to be pampered and loved: Self-care technique is about allowing yourself to be pampered a little bit while pregnant. Allow yourself to feel loved. This could mean going out and getting your hair restyled. It could mean getting a pedicure and manicure done. It could mean an all out "spa day" including a massage and facial. As a pregnant mother you should treat yourself to one spa day a month if possible. Doula Tip: If you have a client that is open to this idea, maybe gift your client a spa day as part of one of your "extra" packages for doula work.

R = Receive, Rejuvenate, relax: Most of the above tips will be helpful for rejuvenating and relaxing. Receiving the right self-care is important. Are you just going out to the spa because your girlfriend insisted, and you would rather go shopping at the mall instead? Make sure you are receiving what you want for self-care. Write down a list of pregnancy things you want to do before baby arrives – you might not get a chance again. Remember to choose a relaxation schedule that works for you. Doula Tip: Remind mother to make a list of pregnancy to do things!

T = Timing of Care, Take Time for yourself, Time for Dad:
This last self-care is to remember to time care right. Perhaps, you are pretty busy and cannot find time for self-care – well, break out a calendar and write in a self-care day. Time for dad – do not forget to include dad in self-care as well. Perhaps, you both can go to the movie together, etc. Think of some self-care things you can both do together as a couple! Doula tip: Remind dad to have some self-care time too!

Unassisted Birth:
We don't recommend mothers to do unassisted birth without a lot of research and knowledge. We also don't recommend it for the first baby, as the experience of having at least one child or labor is better for an unassisted birth. Unassisted birth is not for everyone. However, as *Comfort in Birth Method practitioner doulas* – we don't see anything wrong with helping a mother as long as you know your role is one of observation and not medical. Knowing how to assist in an emergency is also important. For instance, a dad may plan to catch the baby if the baby is coming super-fast before an emergency medical team can arrive. However, some dads will freeze up at the very moment of someone needing to catch the baby. Then it is OK to step in as a doula and make sure the baby doesn't hit the cement or ground and get hurt! We are definitely not advocating that you take the place of a midwife at all. Your role should remain doula if an emergency comes up. (See emergency chapter for more information). Also, to protect yourself legally, you may want to check with your state on what is allowed in case of an emergency or if your state has any information on unassisted birthing. Most likely more of your clients are going to have a midwife on hand or doctor! As a doula you should be prepared for any situation!

If a mother wants to have unassisted birth, come up with a list of questions that you might ask them to better understand her situation. Here are a few examples to start.

Why are you choosing unassisted birth?
What do you wish to see out of this labor and birth?
What do you expect out of my role as your Comfort in Birth Practitioner?
Do you have a support team?
Is everyone who plans to attend supportive of the choice?
Do you plan to complete your own prenatal care? Are you going to work with a doctor or midwife for prenatal care?
What are your thoughts on vaccines, circumcision, and breastfeeding?

Get a feel of her desires and views. After your consultation, think about the conversation and decide if she is a good fit. Wait for her to reach out to you, be sure she has your contact information.

If she hires you to come to an unassisted birth, she may need to convey her desires for her birth to you.

Here are a few examples:
Do you prefer hands-off or physical touch support?
What supplies have you bought/still need to buy?
Is there anything you plan to monitor during labor?
What did you want to be documented? (When transition begins, when baby crowns, when the head is born, what the baby is completely born, and so on)
Do you have a photographer? Would you like me to take photos when possible?
Who will be present for labor and delivery?
Will children be present?
What are the plans for delivery? Who is to "catch" baby? (Mom, dad, child, etc.)
What are your plans for the placenta?

Ask for Quiz over this chapter and turn into instructor!

CHAPTER 15: LABOR POSITIONS, CHALLENGES OF BIRTH & EMERGENCY BIRTH

Comfort in Birth Method™ includes labor positions that will make birth more comfortable to the mother and rebozo techniques to help. We already covered some positions earlier in the stages of labor – showing some pushing positions. Challenges of labor and birth will be included in this section. Emergency birth will be covered just in case you need to help mother during such a situation. Our goal for Comfort in Birth Method™ is to have the mom gain confidence in natural birth setting; however, as we said in beginning, we do support and advocate for what the mother wishes during her birth time. By the way, this section is meant for you to think through and research. So, some of below you will find your own answers and learn by researching the topics. We will briefly cover movement with epidural since we feel that this is an important subject matter and universal precautions at birth. We are expanding this edition of the manual; so, we will include a little bit more information just in case you are at different style birthing situations. Let's talk about positions first!

Labor positions

In this section we want you to explore the terms more – this means research below and find out more about each word or term for labor positioning:

Lunge
Sitting
Swaying or Dancing
Side-Lying

Squat
Hands and Knees
Leaning and or Semi-supported
Double Hip-Squeeze
Counter Pressure
Birth Ball
Peanut Ball

How are lunges done? "A lunge can refer to any position of the human body where one leg is positioned forward with knee bent and foot flat on the ground while the other leg is positioned behind."[lxviii]

<u>How to use the lunge technique:</u> The mother should face forward; the chair or stool is near her side, not in front of her. The mom hangs on to the back of the chair or her support person (husband/doula). The person may stand in front of mom for eye contact support. Mom foot should be flat on the chair. During a "pressure wave" (contraction), mom will rock towards her knee and back to standing up straight again. She will repeat through each "pressure wave." She should try to breathe deeply and slowly as much as possible. She should relax her belly, buttocks, shoulders, etc. She should not extend past her knees. She can rock gently towards the knee and away – much like a *"fencer*

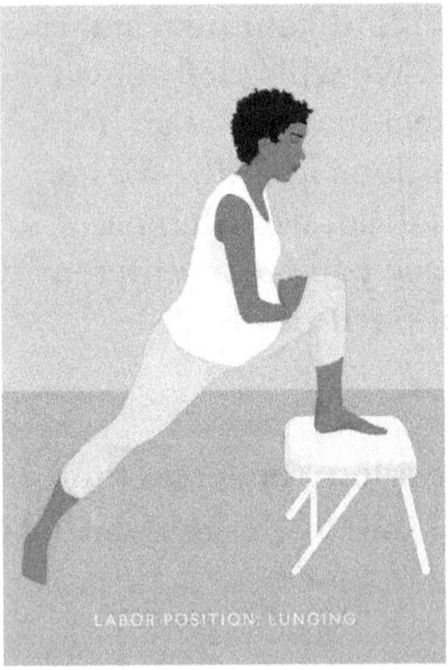

lunging towards an opponent."[lxix] In between "pressure waves", her foot down, rest her knee, and move her legs for circulation. Repeat for 10-20 pressure waves (contractions) – switching legs for better results. Her partner/husband/father or doula can help hold her up for better balance and comfort – so basically this is your job if helping with lunges. "Lifting one leg to open that side of the mid-pelvis makes more room between the ischial spines, or the narrowest part of the interior pelvic passage. Lifting one leg up on a chair opens the mid-pelvis even more, but any amount of lift can be a good thing."[lxx] Direct quotes from spinning babies – rest in our own words.

Why use a lunge at birth? "The Lunge opens the mid-pelvis. It is a good technique to be used in labor during a contraction. Lunges help:

- An **occiput posterior** baby rotate or descend
- An **asynclitic baby** descend
- Overcome a **stall in active labor**."[lxxi]

Sitting positions for birth include:

1. Toilet sitting: This position can be assumed as the name would suggest or with some variations. The mother can sit facing the tank so a birth companion can rub her back or apply counter pressure. If needed, her feet can be supported with low stools to open the pelvis further.
2. Reclined sitting: These modified positions usually involve pillows or other such supports. They are beneficial for complete relaxation. Using a recliner is the most obvious choice. If one is not available, then a wall or even a birthing pool can become options.

3. **Rocking chairs: Using a rocking chair can be one of the most comforting sitting position. It allows the mother to use rhythmic movement to regulate her breathing as well as encouraging the progression of labor. She is also able to fully extend her legs and experiment with different speeds of movement during and between contractions. Source:** https://www.givingbirthnaturally.com/sitting-positions.html

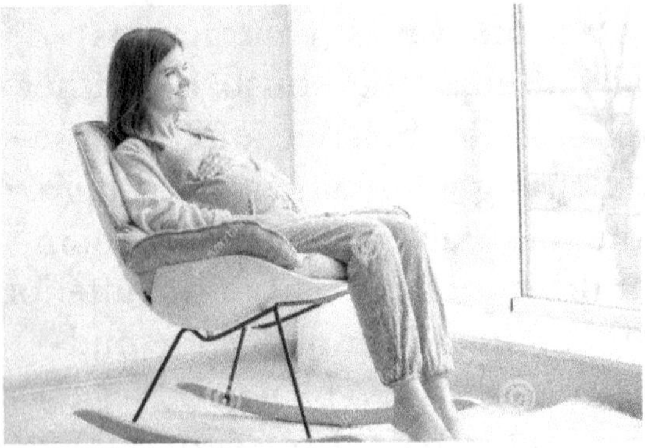

4. ***Dancing or Swaying for birth:***

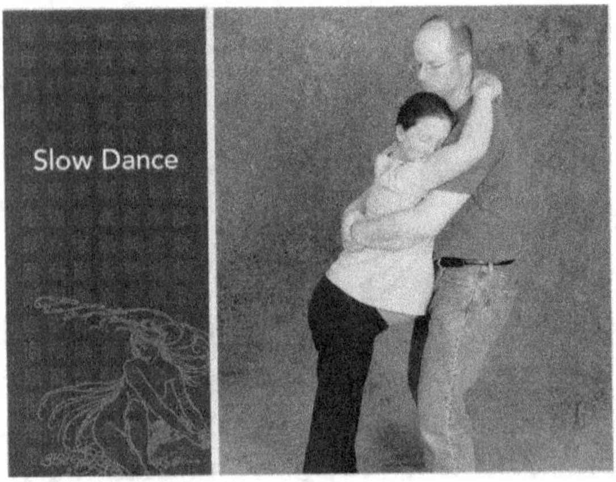

Well, there is a movement called *Dance for Birth*; so, we are going to get information from the founder Stephanie Larson.

Side-lying position

When using a side lying position during labor or for the pushing stage, the mother will rest on one side, with her body slightly curled, or in the "fetal" position (pun intended). (Quote from Birthing naturally)
https://www.givingbirthnaturally.com/side-lying.html

Squats for birthing or the dangle:

In this video Lynn shows two types of squatting for birth:

Video about squatting:

https://www.youtube.com/watch?v=rod23BYjto8

Squatting at birth is like the most natural way to go – this is ancient history. Women have given birth squatting for centuries.

What is the "dangle" position? Article below by a Midwife:

The dangle position is an upright supported squat, which allows the labor partner to support the mother without straining his or her back.

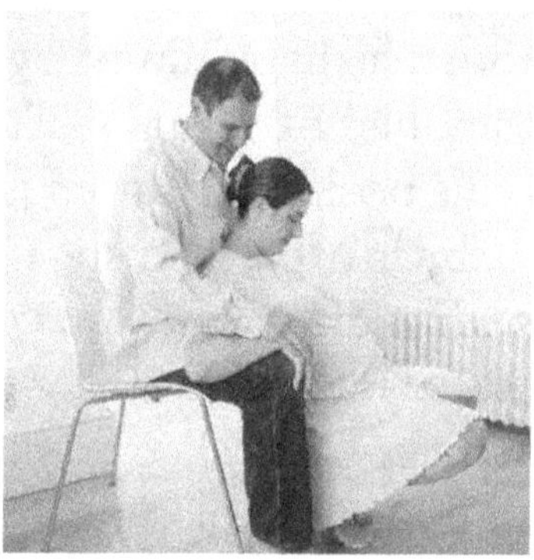

How it works:

Squatting positions take advantage of gravity to increase the work done during contractions. Squatting also widens the outlet of the pelvis, making it easier for the baby to move down.

By stretching the mother's trunk, the dangle increases the room for the baby to move, which may be beneficial if the baby is not sitting well on the cervix (asynclitic). It also gives the mother freedom to move her pelvis while squatting, which further improves the baby's ability to get into an optimal position.

One great benefit to the dangle position is that it is easier on the labor partner than other supported squat positions.

When to do it:

This position can be used when the mother is pushing, or any time in labor when the mother wants to remain upright to encourage process but wants help supporting her body weight.

Incorporating it into labor:

If the mother is fully dilated and not yet feeling an urge to push, the dangle position may help align the baby to begin the pushing reflex. If the mother is experiencing a backache, the dangle position may allow the baby to move relieving the backache. At home, try the dangle in the kitchen, sitting on the counter; in a hospital, try the dangle by raising the bed as high as it will go. Article from: https://psamidwife.com/2016/11/27/labor-positions-the-dangle/

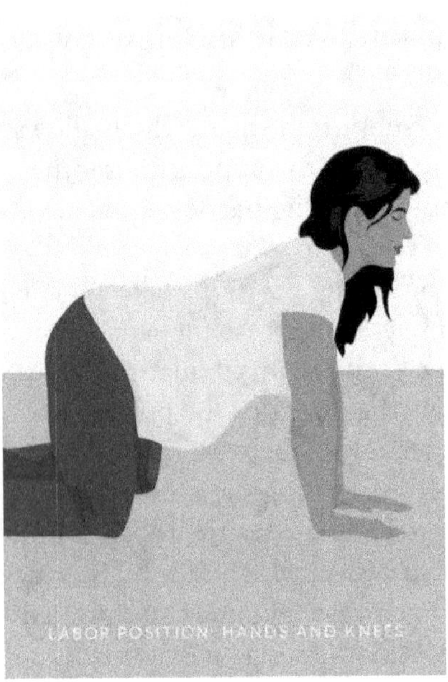

Hands and Knees position is good for pushing.

This can also be used with a rebozo for sifting. See rebozo section. The baby can be repositioned by sifting while mom is in this position. If mom is feeling like baby is off – then she may want to try this. Make sure you consult doctor or midwife if doing this before labor time. We do not know about things like placenta separation, etc. If mom is having placenta issues, she should always consult doctor or midwife.

We already covered some about birth ball and peanut ball – please go back to that section if you want to re-study that. Also, you can take our Royal Rebozo Way Level B for more on birth ball.

Enrichment Handout Exercise: **Make a handout about the above labor positions. Turn in your handout for credit for the course.**

More about Squats (Extra bonus):

Squatting is an important exercise for mothers to try and use during pregnancy. Squats will help the mother's pelvis open up and make labor easier for the mother. So, a mother should be doing several squats a day. We will share some videos and links to this in our "module" portion of our class. If you are a mom reading this – we suggest looking at YouTube for videos on squatting.

Get into Rhythm and birth! One of the challenges of labor is that the mother loses her rhythm during childbirth. She may become a bit tired, exhausted, etc. Using rhythm techniques will help the mother establish a way to overcome this challenge of labor. Now, this does not mean we will not listen to the doctor. If the doctor or midwife is calling for a procedure – remember to use the B.R.A.I.N. formula as mentioned before. Perhaps, the doctor wants to try Pitocin to get the labor going a bit faster. Perhaps, the midwife wants to break the waters. Just remember B.R.A.I.N. too!

Usually at birth, the mother will be able to establish a rhythm during labor. This usually involves proper breathing techniques, relaxation techniques, and helping mom stay strong through surges (contractions). Penny Simkin is my favorite for her methods on showing you how to do this rhythmic movements during labor. She talks about Rhythm, relaxation, and ritual.

Relaxation: According to Penny Simkin, the first step is relaxation to help mom during labor. The mother needs to try to completely relax in between contractions—try to go limp like a "ragdoll" kitty cat and just focus on breathing deeply and fully. This will help release tension and the pregnant mother will be able to cope better with the coming contractions. **"Alternatively, it is also soothing and relaxing to sway, rock, moan, chant, or sing rhythmically. This is called 'active relaxation' and can be helpful, especially with intense contractions of later labor, or if passive relaxation is no longer doable."[lxxii]**

Rhythmic movements help reduce anxiety and pain.

Walking, rocking, and swaying help self-soothe the mother.

Rhythmic breathing helps the mother cope better with the pain.

Rhythmic massage or touch with essential oils (aromatherapy) can help the mother cope better.

Empowering verbalizations can help the mother have "verbal anesthesia"—praise is always good for a mother to hear.

Music and slow dancing can help.

Chanting can help—we recommend "Jesus have mercy" or some type of Christian/Catholic "mantra".

Deep vocalization coming from the chest.

Ritual can mean various things to mothers. If a mother is Jewish as mentioned earlier, the mother needs to not have a man nearby for her birth. Another mother may have ritual of having a sister or relative nearby for her birth time. We already discussed some birth traditions, so those would follow under ritual.

Enrichment activity E for mothers: Mothers may want to explore the full Penny Simkin website at www.pennysimkin.com and go to the resources link. She has many videos and handouts that you can look up items that may fit if you are having challenges such as breech baby, and things like that.

Enrichment activity for students: We would like you to consider working with a mother on a practice "Take Charge Routine" for her labor time. Ask an instructor if you need more help. Read this handout link:
https://www.dancingstarbirth.ca/Handouts/Take_Charge_Routine.pdf

Epidurals and movement:

Many mothers like to get an epidural for birth. It appeals to them. It means they will not have "pain" during labor. Or some mothers have little tolerance for pain. There are some tools that you can use to help a mother know what she can tolerate during labor or not. We are not going to cover that so much. Most mothers will know whether or not they wish to experience natural labor or not.

Extra information: Having an epidural does not mean the mother will experience no pain – it only means she will have less pain. Some epidurals do not take as well for some mothers as others.

Occasionally an epidural will only numb like the left side or right side of the body. A mother can request a "lighter" epidural if she wants to have more ability to control her pushing stage.

Research time: Doulas and mamas both should understand the whole epidural procedure. (We will put more information in our formal modules).

Question: What does it take to have an epidural? What medications are used?

We want you to research this on your own! Write a short paragraph on what you learned.

Movement and epidurals. Recently, more evidence shows that a mother can move "very carefully" when she has an epidural. She will need assistance moving to like a hands and knees position on the bed or possibly leaning on a birth ball in bed. Ask the nurses if they can try turning mother over. If they cannot do a full turn around, at least see if they will consider having mother use a peanut ball. This article explains the use of peanut balls in depth: https://premierbirthtools.com/peanut-balls-for-labor/

Question: Research further – Can a mother move around with an epidural? Can she use a peanut ball to help? What did you find out? What is your local hospitals procedure?

Question: How can a birth ball be used during labor (for more natural birth or before an epidural is given)?

Universal Procedures and emergency birth:

Universal precautions mean that we take extra measures not to get into contact with certain fluids from the mother or blood if possible. However, sometimes the unavoidable happens. So, a doula should probably "glove up" during a birth if possible. We think it is important to know if a client has HIV, STD, etc. If so, the doula can take better precautions to avoid fluids from the client. Here's a link to an article that would be a good one to read further: https://www.inspiredbirthpro.com/doula-prevent-spread-sexually-transmitted-infections-on-job/

It is also important as a doula to have a "uniform" that you wish to use during birth or delivery of the baby. If you use the same clothes for births, then you will have a professional status. Mothers may feel safer if you have gloves on. *Wearing a mask is an extra precaution you can also consider.*

Challenges of Labor Section:

Emergency birth. As a doula, it is not in our scope of practice to act like a doctor or midwife. However, in an emergency situation, mothers may need an extra calm person to be there and help get things situated even if a doctor, nurse or ER is coming over. The doula can help ease the mother into a relaxed state and she may be able to birth unassisted if need be or perhaps assisted by her husband/partner. A doula can call 9-1-1 for the mother to ask for assistance. The doula can prepare a safe landing space for the baby. The doula should help guide the mother through her surges (contractions) just like she would do regularly. The doula should guide the mother to "catch" her own baby or get husband/partner to assist if no one has arrived yet. The doula should not do anything medical. She should not do any cervical checks, blood pressure checks, etc. Let the birthing process come naturally. The cord should not be cut unless the cord is wrapped tightly around the baby's neck – then in that case the cord should be quickly cut if need be. The preference would be to unwrap cord and let it stop pulsating naturally while help arrives.

Challenges of Birth/Labor – Placenta Previa:

Placenta Previa information from American pregnnacy[lxxiii]:

Placenta Previa is a condition where the placenta lies low in the uterus and partially or completely covers the cervix. The placenta may separate from the uterine wall as the cervix begins to dilate (open) during labor.

How Common Is Placenta Previa?

Placenta previa affects about 1 in 200 pregnant women in the third trimester of pregnancy.

It is more common in women who have had one or more of the following:
More than one child
A cesarean birth
Surgery on the uterus
Twins or triplets

What Are the Different Types?
Complete Previa: the cervical opening is completely covered
Partial Previa: a portion of the cervix is covered by the placenta
Marginal Previa: extends just to the edge of the cervix

What Are the Symptoms?

Signs and symptoms may vary, but the most common symptom is painless bleeding during the third trimester.

Other Signs and Symptoms Include:
Premature contractions
Baby is breech, or in a transverse position
Uterus measures larger than it should according to gestational age.

Once diagnosed, treatment will usually include bed rest for the mother and frequent hospital visits. Depending on the gestational age, steroid shots may be given to help mature the baby's lungs. If the mother experiences bleeding that cannot be controlled, immediate cesarean delivery is usually done regardless of the length of the pregnancy. Some marginal previas can be delivered vaginally, although complete or partial previas would require a cesarean delivery.

Most physicians will also recommend limiting the following activities:

Avoid intercourse
Limit traveling
Avoid pelvic exams

- *Risks: If over the age of 35*
- *Had more than four pregnancies*
- *Have a history of uterine surgery (regardless of incision type)*

Placenta previa usually can be diagnosed with an ultrasound and a c-section is usually the best answer to this unless the placenta moves out of the way.

Enrichment Activity F: Research the terms – give definitions for all listed.

Message teacher with 3 types of placenta previa.

Submit to instructor @ comfortinbirth@gmail.com

Breech Babies:

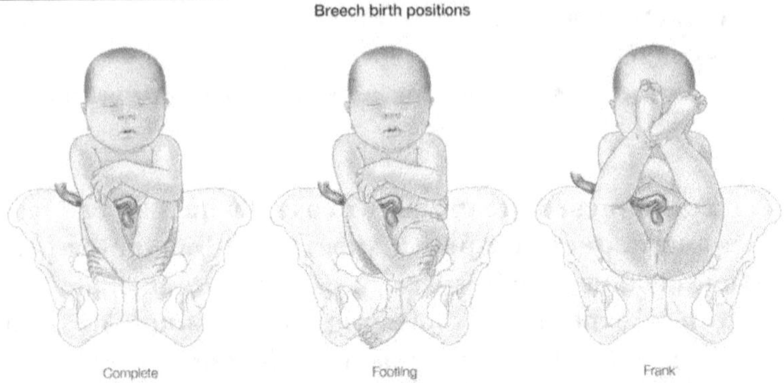

There's 3-4 types of breech births. There's the complete breech, incomplete includes footling breech and some rare instances of baby kneeling inside the mother, and there's also the frank breech. (See above pictures of 3 types).

In order to understand breech babies better we have a research assignment below. What if a mother wants a natural breech birth? It is possible! A mother will most likely need to seek out a midwife who will perform a breech as most regular doctors are just not well versed in it.

Research assignment: Go to spinning babies website: www.spinningbabies.com and research breech births.

Here are some articles from them to help:

1. https://www.spinningbabies.com/pregnancy-birth/baby-position/breech/when-is-breech-an-issue/
2. https://www.spinningbabies.com/pregnancy-birth/techniques/other-techniques/breech-tilt/
3. https://www.spinningbabies.com/pregnancy-birth/baby-position/breech/breech-for-providers/

What techniques that are natural that can help a breech baby turn?

Ask for quiz for this module.

Cord Prolapse – what is it and what to do – emergency situation!

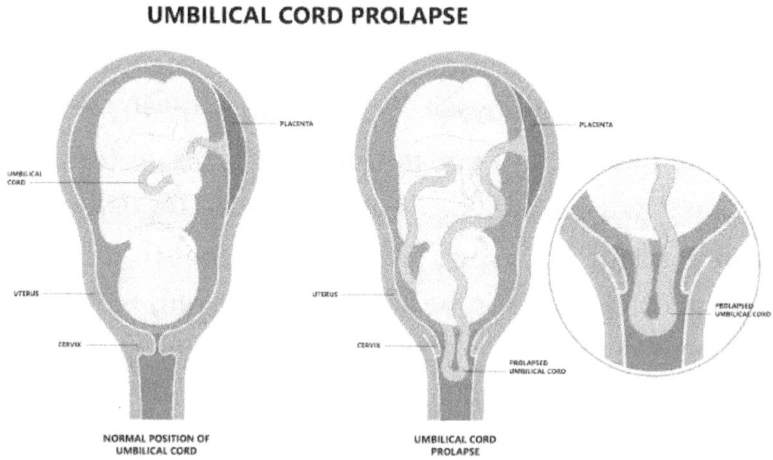

Cord prolapse is when the cord comes down before the baby's head and basically blocks the passageway for baby. Usually, the cord is above the baby's head and will not get in the way. Also, sometimes the cord is wrapped around the baby's neck. This does not mean the child cannot be born. For instance, my first child was born at home and her cord was wrapped around her neck, the midwife quickly unwrapped the cord – and I was none the wiser about the situation (till hubby told me later!) The cord is the lifeline of the baby – it gives the baby all his/her nutrients and oxygen. So, having a cord prolapse is a dangerous situation. Doctor or ER personnel should handle this. However, for emergency birth reasons, we include information on how a doula can be helpful. If the mother looks like she is going to have that baby "right now" and the cord is showing instead of a head, first of all a doula should call 9-1-1. Get information over the phone as you wait for help to arrive.

Doula Tip to help: If mother is having issues with cord prolapse – try the following: Mother should try the "Miles Circuit" pose or knees to chest. Watch this video for more ideas: https://www.youtube.com/watch?v=WQUhdWtd1ao

As you wait for ER crew, try to get mother to relax, remember you are there to be her "calm" among any storm!

Quiz over this chapter: Email instructor for quiz. Thank you.

CHAPTER 16: VBAC Section

VBAC – a Vaginal birth after cesarean is sometimes not that easy to obtain. Some mothers will not even seek this; other mothers were not told that it is possible. Doulas should be well-versed or have knowledge that this can be a possibility for low-risk mothers. Even a medium risk mom may still have a chance at a VBAC. A mother first needs to know and want this for herself. As a doula you are an advocate, but if the mother does not want a VBAC, there is nothing you can do about it. This is her decision and her body. Make the best of another C-section if you are helping a mom with one.

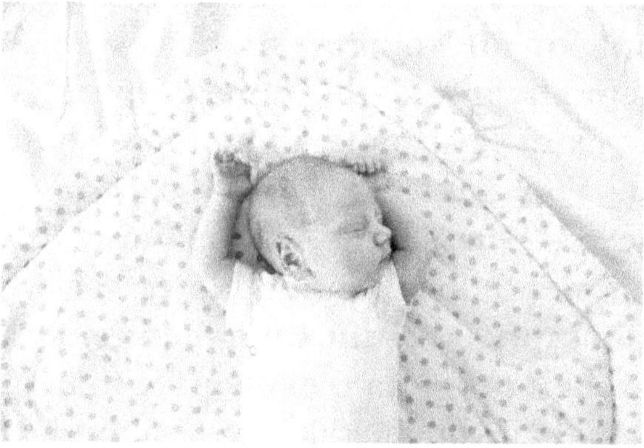

Seven Tips to help moms that want a VBAC[lxxiv] by Julie Larsen:

1. Labor at home as long as possible. Here's some more tips at this website: https://www.motherrisingbirth.com/2016/10/tips-for-a-successful-vbac.html Laboring at home longer can make the difference between a VBAC vs. C-section. The mother should wait till she is in transition to head to hospital. (If she is close enough to the hospital to do this). Also, a

mother may want to consider a home VBAC – that way she does not have to travel to have the baby.

2. Have a doctor that is willing to do a VBAC or Home VBAC. A lot of midwives can offer a VBAC and may have more experience than a doctor (OB). Ask how much experience your provider has in this situation?
3. Make sure mother has all the research she needs. Get her over to Evidence Based Birth website www.evidencebasedbirth.com and www.mamanatural.com are good sites to look at.
4. The mother should hire a doula! Tell her doulas can help her be able to have a healthier and longer natural labor. Be honest with mom if this is your first VBAC – tell her this is my first one, but you are going to be the best possible anchor for this mother to get this done properly. You may want to take an extra class on learning more about VBAC. https://www.thevbaclink.com/vbac-doula-training/ We may offer some extra class in this in the future; but for now, we highly recommend this training. Note: You will need to contact them about their certification requirements, etc. And the cost of their program maybe more than our class even! So, it depends if you feel like this training will help you get more births or clients!
5. The mother may need to be willing to switch providers mid-way through her pregnancy. If a provider is going to recommend or make the mother have an induction by a certain point in time; the mother may need to switch to someone else.
6. The mother may need to consider even an unassisted birth! There are midwives that offer midwifery services up to 40 weeks or 42 weeks. After that, they have to stop because of regulations of their state. If your mother is a type that has

gone past her due date in the past, then she may need to consider unassisted birth! A doula, if she goes to an unassisted birth, must not practice as a doula but be an observer only. Some doulas will not go to an unassisted birth while others will do so. We encourage you to do what you feel comfortable doing. Our scope of practice does not forbid you attending unassisted births as long as you are practicing as a doula! See previous section about unassisted birth.

7. **The mother needs to know this is "her body, her birth". Whatever decisions she makes for her VBAC – you are there to support her even if the VBAC does not work out and she needs a repeat emergency C-section – you are that rock this mother needs. Celebrate the birth of her child with her!**

<u>Further Reading</u> for mothers or yourself about VBAC. We highly recommend if you want to know more about VBAC to read up on it – here is a book list:

- <u>Brave Beautiful Birth: Trusting God Through VBAC</u> Paperback – August 8, 2018 by Jaimie M. Schrock (This book might be also good if you are doing the PEACE project and looking for something for "Allowing God into the Birth room."
- <u>Give Birth a Chance: How to Prepare for an Empowered VBAC</u> Paperback – February 20, 2018 by Ilia Blandina CNM
- <u>Birth Without Fear: The Judgment-Free Guide to Taking Charge of Your Pregnancy, Birth, and Postpartum</u> Paperback – March 5, 2019 by January Harshe
- <u>Silent Knife: Cesarean Prevention and Vaginal Birth after Cesarean (VBAC)</u> by Lois J Estner
- <u>Cut, Stapled, and Mended: When One Woman Reclaimed Her Body and Gave Birth on Her Own Terms After Cesarean</u> Paperback – May 14, 2013 by Roanna Rosewood

- The VBAC Companion: The Expectant Mother's Guide to Vaginal Birth After Cesarean (Non) Paperback – November 19, 1997 by Diana Korte
- **Home Birth On Your Own Terms: A How To Guide For Birthing Unassisted** Kindle Edition by Heather Baker – A mother may want to read up on unassisted birth.
- ***Freebirth - Self-Directed Pregnancy and Birth*** Paperback – March 27, 2015 by Sarah Schmid
- ***Unassisted Childbirth, 2nd Edition:*** by Laura Shanley
- ***Fearless Birthing: Clear Your Fears for a Positive Birth*** by Alexia Leachman
- ***Please choose one of these books as a book review for this course if taking our class for certification purposes!***

Links to some articles to read further about VBAC and videos – note these were working at time of printing this:

- https://www.romper.com/p/how-to-naturally-induce-labor-for-a-vbac-avoid-induction-9801239
- https://www.thevbaclink.com/how-to-have-a-successful-vbac/
- https://onestrongmama.com/preparing-for-a-successful-vbac-birth/
- https://thesnapmom.com/17-tips-for-a-successful-vbac/
- https://www.youtube.com/watch?v=bgAK_hMWXSY
- https://www.youtube.com/watch?v=gADqJrpdgYQ
- https://www.youtube.com/watch?v=a1UyhTuiyEg
- https://www.youtube.com/watch?v=Gvi1lw6wgZI **(Once a C-section always a C-section – why this is wrong!)**
- https://www.youtube.com/watch?v=pFH880bEuIo (African American mother)
- https://www.youtube.com/watch?v=dRcOBoSI-Ks (African American mother)
- https://www.youtube.com/watch?v=YoZ1fyFDcTQ (Goode, Bad, Ugly)

- <u>Assignment for students of Comfort in Birth™ students:</u>
- Please read one article above or book and summarize it and turn it into instructor.
- Please watch one video and summarize what you learned and turn into instructor. Also, on the video – would you recommend a mother to watch? What did you like about the video? What did you not like? (If anything), etc. Write it like an amazon review – with 5 stars being super great!

Chapter 17: HOSPITAL TO HOME: BABY IS HERE!

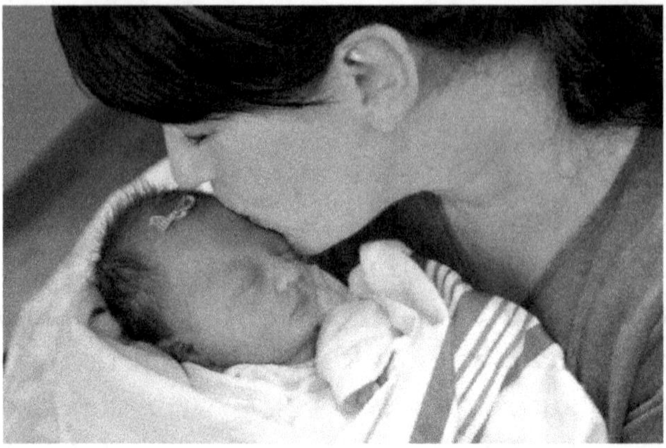

Signs of labor: It is important to know the signs of labor for mother before she wants to head to hospital or birth center. Is she really in labor or just early warning signs?

One of the signs of labor that is pretty obvious is losing the mucus plug. This plug kind of keeps the cervix in place and when the plug comes out – there is this "bloody show" that comes forth and the mother may also start to feel a bit crampy like a period. The mother should not worry too much. This is a sign that the baby is coming soon. Sometimes the mother will go into labor within 24 hours of "bloody show" while other mothers it might still be a week.

"Baby drops" this one will usually happen a few weeks before labor begins. The baby usually will drop his head and body more into the pelvis region. Usually your heartburn will not be as bad (for mother).

"Cervix dilates" – this is pretty obvious – the cervix will start dilating and opening up more when baby is getting engaged to come down the canal! A doctor or midwife can usually check to see what dilation mom is at before labor begins. Some mothers will be at 1-3 cm even before surges (contractions) begin.

"Nesting syndrome" – I really like this one. I usually would have this nesting syndrome around 2 weeks before the baby came. I would start organizing my house more, getting the baby area or room ready. One time I went shopping for baby things and I went into labor *literally the next day*!

"You feel stronger frequent contractions" – This is different than Braxton-Hicks. The Braxton-hicks kind of surges usually are sporadic and do not make sense to anyone. One of my last pregnancies, I kept on getting the Braxton-hicks at bedtime when I wanted to lay down – they would literally kick in. It made bedtime kind of hard; I had to find a way to kind of sit up and sleep! *Real contractions will have a reason and rhythm to them for the most part*!

I hope this mini guide to pre-labor signs will help you as a mother or doula. If you see bloody show, that would be a good time to call your doctor or midwife and discuss any further steps with them. If you feel regular surges, then you may want to get out a contraction timer online or your phone and see how far apart they are and go from there on calling the doctor or midwife! Remember most midwives do not mind false alarms!

We are going to cover some more terms in this section. You get to explore them and that way you are doing some action and research. If taking for certification, please send terms to instructor.

Hospital Procedure Terms

Electrical Fetal monitoring
Internal Fetal monitoring
IV (IV fluids)

Pitocin
Cervidil
C-Section
VBAC
Drugs commonly used at labor
Oxygen
Epidural – define, explain procedure
Catheter
Forceps
Vacuum Extraction
Cord Clamping
Breastfeeding
Kangaroo Care
Vitamin K shot
Jaundice
Vaccinations
Eye ointment

Inductions for Birth/Labor

We really do not consider Inductions part of "Comfort in Birth method" as we are aiming for clients to go naturally; however, we accept that inductions are being done every day and doulas need to know about them.

An induction is an artificial means of getting labor started and hopefully continuing labor till the baby comes out. However, sometimes the induction does not work and puts mother at risk for infection or baby might go into distress and mom will end up with a C-section birth.

□ There are "two" types of inductions—natural induction methods and non-natural (medicated) induction.

□ It is also important that the mother know her "Bishop's score" before she makes a decision on an induction procedure or not.

What is a Bishop's score? It is a way of measuring the location of the baby inside the mother as well as obtaining information if mom is dilating or not. It is important because if baby is in a higher up position then an induction may not really work. Here is an article about "bishop's score": http://www.amazingpregnancy.com/pregnancy-articles/173-html.html

□ A score of "5" or less is supposed to mean "unfavorable" for an induction at that time. Mom may need to persuade her care provider to wait a week or two to try induction at a better time frame.

Self-help induction methods (natural):

- Nipple stimulation (massage, breast pump, breastfeeding)
- Walking (going for walk can get labor moving)
- Acupressure or Acupuncture (if a mother knows a person that can do this – most likely done before going to hospital).
- Castor oil (should only be done with medical supervision of doctor or midwife – this can turn south easy).
- "Oxytocin – natural way (ie: sex)" – should only be done if person is married ☺
- Teas, tinctures, herbs, etc. (Consult a midwife on right herbs for this).

Discussion Question: Do you think self-induction methods work? Support your argument with an article from the Internet. Please list the source. Submit to instructor.

Medical inductions:

1. "Stripping the Membranes"
2. AROM (we already covered)

3. Prostaglandin gels: Prepidil or Cervidil may be used. Cytotec is also sometimes used but this is more dangerous and can lead to baby dying – not recommended.
4. Pitocin can be used for induction. This is synthetic Oxytocin.
5. Read about pros vs. cons of inductions: https://health.usnews.com/health-news/news/articles/2012/05/11/induced-labor-late-in-pregnancy-has-pros-cons
6. Read this Mayo Clinic article – it suggests that inductions should not be before 39 weeks pregnancy: https://www.mayoclinic.org/healthy-lifestyle/labor-and-delivery/in-depth/inducing-labor/art-20047557
7. Read this article about Big babies: http://evidencebasedbirth.com/evidence-for-induction-or-c-section-for-big-baby

More about Monitoring mother in the hospital from monitoring to epidurals!

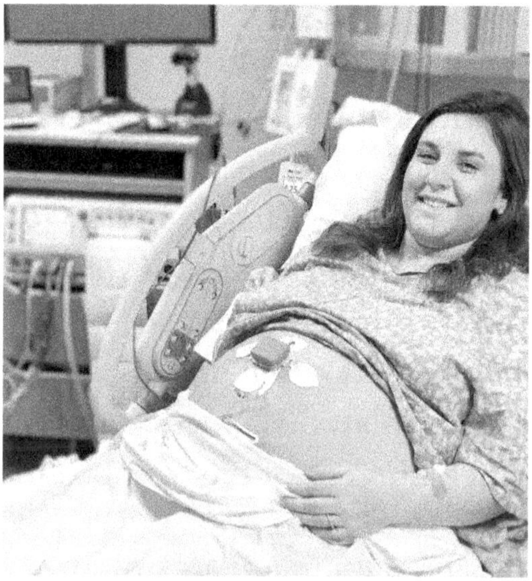

Once the mother is in the "room" – out come the Electric Fetal Monitoring devices (two belts that go around your lap).

They may also take your blood pressure, temperature, etc.

They also draw blood for tests esp. if you are a last-minute patient.

Alternative? Let them do the EFM once and then say: "I want to disconnect this and be monitored by a Doppler every 15-20 minutes, so I can have more freedom of movement in labor." This sometimes works depending on your agreement with doctor or midwife beforehand. However, most hospitals are going to want to tie you down every 20-30 minutes on the monitor and then you can go for a walk or something.

- A mother is sometimes automatically put on a water IV—which is technically sugar water. This can lead to issues of edema. You need to find out if you can refuse this type of IV and ask to just be given plenty of fluids to drink. IV's give a false sense of fluids in the body during labor.
- Antibiotics for GBS will be put in mother usually in form of an IV; so in this case that is a necessary evil. Arrive early

enough to get the IV over with and not hopefully have to do 2. (Sometimes they will do a second one if baby is not born 4 hours later). If you don't have any idea – try to just get their early or try to have mom checked at 36 weeks for this. A mother is sometimes automatically put on a water IV—which is technically sugar water. This can lead to issues of edema. You need to find out if you can refuse this type of IV and ask to just be given plenty of fluids to drink. IV's give a false sense of fluids in the body during labor.

◦ Forceps are rarely used these days but are still available. Vacuum extraction is where they place like suction cup on the baby's head and try to suck him out of the womb. This can be an alternative to a C-section.

◦ Vacuum extraction does come in handy if a mother is struggling to push baby out and the head is right there.

◦ Epidurals are quite common; a mother that you are working with may request this. So, unless she wants to consider natural birth as an "alternative" then she will most likely proceed with it. Video of epidural: https://www.youtube.com/watch?v=IMVLr9Z4XFU

◦ If your mother is uncertain before birth whether she wants an epidural, then that is the time to influence her; but once she is in labor this is the time to support her decision on having one. Remember this so she will know that she hired the right doula! Video of an epidural: https://www.youtube.com/watch?v=3PzQyqW-3a4

◦ As a doula, you are there to support the mom's choice even for an epidural. However, a mother should consider the words of B.R.A.I.N. and determine if the pros vs. cons outweigh each other.

- Find 3 resources to kind of get mom to at least consider changing her mind. Make a handout from your 3 resources (Can be a book, Internet, Journal article, Midwifery Today, etc.) Submit "Epidural Handout" to instructor.
-
- Write up 3 things you learned from the above section as well and submit them to your instructor for the class.

When mom is in labor and she may change her mind at the hospital about having an epidural or medicines, it is good idea to come up with a "code word" for mom to use. That way if she says "I want an epidural or pain medicine" then the husband or family member or doula can know that she's not really serious. But if mom says the "code word" like "peanut butter" then the family member knows she serious. Code word for mom is a good idea to have written also in the birth plan when working with your doula client. Extra Credit: Make up your own code word for labor just in case you need one!

Baby Procedures at hospital:

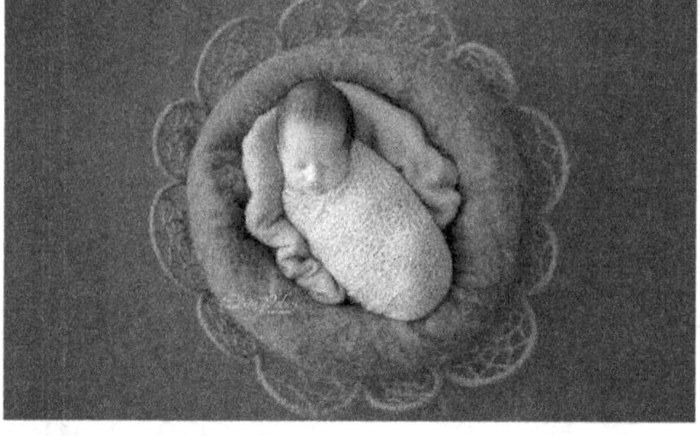

Be aware of hospital procedures during labor and for the baby. There are times when you may have to let the hospital staff do their business even if you do not agree exactly because they are going to anyway! So, for example, if a baby is born and is not responding so well, the nurses will probably help the doctor get the cord cut quickly and pat down baby and get the baby breathing fast. At a home birth this would be done in a different way with the midwife probably keeping the cord attached and try suctioning first. So, anyway, there are different methods for hospital and home birth. Nowadays there might be more opportunities for helping at a home birth.

Baby Procedures to study:

Hepatitis B Vaccine: Cons – this vaccine is done unnecessarily as there is little chances for most women to be carries of Hepatitis. Also, why a vaccine at birth? Just more trauma for an infant.

Eye Ointment for baby: Pros: If mother has a STD, supposed to help stop any infection on baby. Cons, if a mother doesn't have this issue, it is almost always done anyway even at homebirths. As a doula you can advocate for the mother and see if she can refuse this procedure. Why put eye ointment on if you are not a carrier? More research needs to be done. Some hospitals still insist on the procedure.

Vitamin K shot: Pros: It can help jaundice in babies. It can help blood clot better. Cons: My first baby had "breastfeeding" jaundice and we did do the Vitamin K shot – so this shot is not full proof on that item. However, evidence for not using Vitamin k is out there. This is something for you to consider researching on your own. You can look at www.evidencebasedbirth.com for a place to explore this topic.

Hearing exam: Pros: Well, it is good to know your baby can hear well. Most of the time this test can be done as they are sleeping and harmless. Cons: It depends on what type of hearing test is done – most of them now are like above and can be done while baby is sleeping. However, if it does something like loud noises, etc. then you may want to reconsider. Ask the doctor what style of test is done for hearing.

PKU test: This is the test where they prick the baby's heel and send it off to lab to determine if baby has other issues that might be of concern. Pro: You get to find out if baby has issues with certain things. Cons: I personally would have preferred this test to be done a few weeks after birth instead of at birth – and I never got the results of any of the ones done – even if they were all negative – it would have been nice to have the information.

Down Syndrome confirmation test:

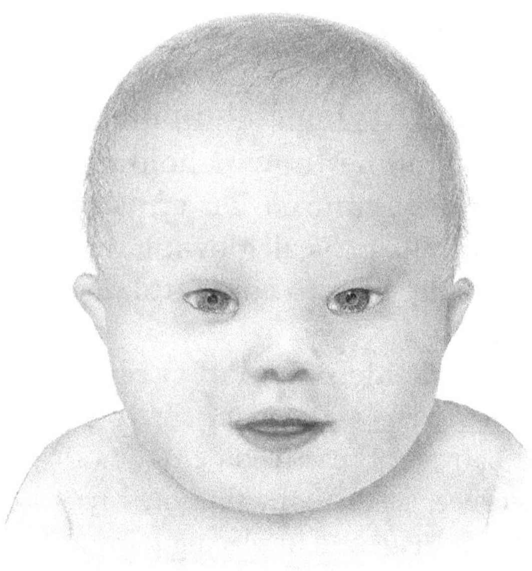

This is also a blood test – should be done if baby looks like he/she has Down Syndrome features or if doctor suspects it. Pros: Parents will have an answer within a week. Cons: The wait for answers – but the staff will usually treat the child as special needs if baby has features of this syndrome. The problem is some children have Mosaic Down Syndrome and don't always have all the features. (Mosaic means a lesser degree). Also, if parents are unsure, they may not know what to ask for at hospital. Parents should still insist on the heart doppler test to see if there are any heart issues with the baby.

Bilirubin Test: To determine if baby has jaundice. Pros: Baby might have this. Cons: Sometimes a baby gets jaundice from breastfeeding (which is a different type). Asking the doctor to let you wait a few days and a retest should be an option. What is done: In hospital, they will put baby under artificial light therapy. At home you could take a baby out in the sun, etc.

Enrichment Activity "M": Find evidence-based articles on one of the procedures for baby above. Write up a short sympnosis of what you found – pros, cons, etc. How common is it that parents can refuse a test? Etc.

Postpartum time and breastfeeding (at hospital).

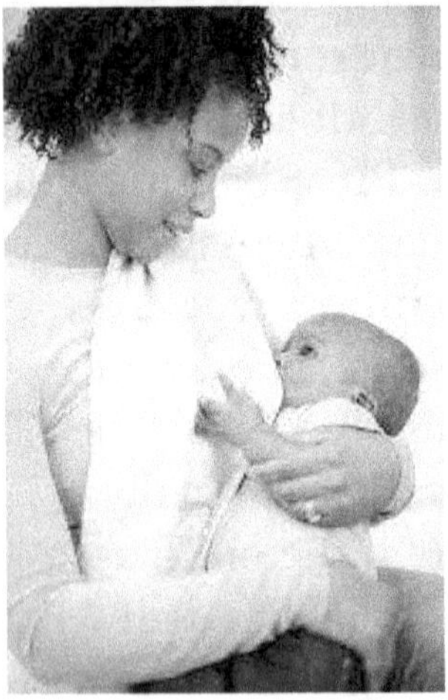

The mother now is holding her baby for the first time in her arms (or at least hopefully)! She is all glowing with "pride." Now is the time to congratulate mom on a good job.

The Golden Hour after birth:
This is a special time – make sure the mother and baby get breastfeeding right away. However, let the baby find the breast himself. Be gentle in placing baby at breast. Sometimes nurses are rough in doing this. **Look up the Thompson Method if you want to know more about Golden Hour.**
https://www.thethompsonmethod.com/

Usually a doula will stay for the first hour after birth! So, the doula needs to do so in order to see about breastfeeding and making sure mom is comfortable with this role. Lactation consultants for staff can still help as needed. If you need to leave earlier, make sure you call back the next morning to see how mom and baby are doing.

Follow up visit:

A doula should follow up one week after birth to see how mom and baby are doing and keep in contact with mom during that time via phone, etc. We will talk more about what to cover in this in the business section.

Postpartum issues

A first-time mother may not know what to expect after postpartum. My mom never told me about "lochia". That is the light bleeding from the uterus that lasts around 6-week time frame. A mother may not know that much about healing after birth. Her bottom may be sore from delivery. She may have had stitches. She needs to know a little more about self-care after birth. She should make sure she has pads on hand to change often. She should have a perineum bottle to use as a spray during first few days after hospital stay – instead of wiping with toilet paper. She should have a padsicle or ice to use for healing. The hospital may send her home with a few things. However, you could make some "homemade" padsicle for instance to give to a client.

> "Homemade Padsicle Recipe from Mama Natural:
> Ingredients:
> 4 tablespoons calendula flower
> 2 tablespoons comfrey leaf
> 2 tablespoons of plantain leaf
> Overnight sanitary pads

Spray bottle
Freezer bag

To make the padsicles: Steep the herbs listed above in a gallon of hot, filtered water for 15-30 minutes.

Strain out the herbs and let the solution cool.

Pour the tea into a spray bottle, then spray a thin, even layer on menstrual pads. (They should feel wet, but not completely saturated.) Fold the pads back into their protective wrapping, place in a freezer bag, and store in the freezer until ready to use."[lxxv]

Explore More: Explore postpartum blues vs. postpartum depression. Write down at least 3 signs of postpartum depression.

1.
2.
3.

Explore More: Breastfeeding can be challenging to some mothers. Write down at least 3 common issues that keep mothers from breastfeeding beyond 6 months.

1.
2.
3.

Please submit sources for the above challenges.

Pushing and pushing with rebozo.

We wanted to add in extra information about pushing techniques. Many mothers have difficulty with this stage of labor because they are not up right, or they are stuck to a bed. So, we want to offer a few tips.

A mother should aim to be in an upright position as much as possible for pushing. Letting Gravity do the work really helps open up the pelvis and allow the baby to move down.

Types of pushing:

Usually if you go to the hospital, they do "direct" pushing. Pushing this way is done by doing "breathe in" and then "count down to 10" as the mother breathes out and pushes at the same time. Now, this type of pushing is not all bad, but it also kind of not helpful if the mother is "holding her breath" as she is pushing. The mother needs to breathe through the whole process. So, if you are a doula and helping with directed pushing; make sure the mother is breathing and not holding her breath!

The second type of pushing is more of a self-directed or let the baby come on down on his own. This is something I think I accomplished or close to it with my third baby as a water birth. I did some blowing technique in between pushing in order to gain some momentum. *This blowing technique is very Ina May Gaskin style!* So, anyway, allowing the baby to come out with natural pushing sometimes works a lot better for mothers. These natural urges should be listened to by the mother and allow her to follow these instincts. I do not like it when doctors say no to push when that is what the mother feels like she needs to do at that instant!

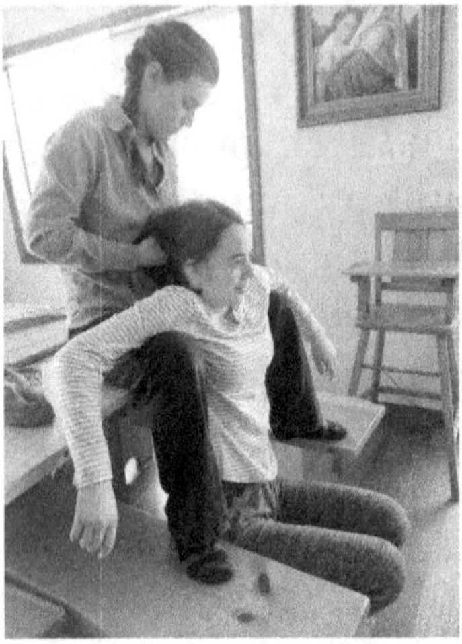

Rebozo can be used for pushing. You can hang the rebozo from a door and allow the mother to hold rebozo as she pushes in a squatting position. The rebozo could be used in the dangle pose to help hold up the mother better for pushing technique. The rebozo can be used other ways as well. (See our mini rebozo booklet).[lxxvi]

Anyway, the pushing styles can vary for a mother and she should be encouraged to seek an upright birth position for her pushing stage in order to ease baby out faster and smoother!

Enrichment "P" Pushing Assignment:

Use the video below:

Pushing by HypnoBirthing:
https://www.youtube.com/watch?v=rcO8sccdk7Y

Practice with a friend the two ways of breathing – like the directed and then the more natural way (breathe as energy).

See how you feel the differences.

Write a paragraph of your practice session and tell us who was your friend that you practiced with. (name can be anonymous if so desired).

Rate your session 1- for not so great to 5-for great learned this well. Submit to comfortinbirth@gmail.com Also, email instructor for quiz over this chapter. Thank you.

CHAPTER 18: HEART OF BUSINESS AND APPLYING COMFORT IN BIRTH ACRONYM TO YOUR WORK!

Welcome to the "heart of business" section. We hope you will learn enough to get started or launched into the "doula world." Please also consider reading "Doing Business the Doula Way" as a way to learn more please contact us for more information about Business classes. Thank you.

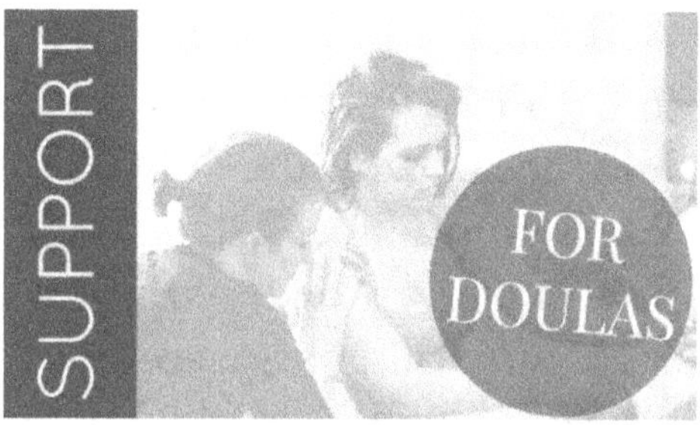

Finding your niche audience – we mentioned this at the very beginning in the introduction letter. That you as a business can be "choosy" about who you want to serve. You do not have to serve every woman you come across. In fact, it is better if you narrow down your spectrum of who you want to serve. So, think about where you go and who you see is pregnant. For instance, if I go to the CrossFit in my town and I see pregnant women working out – this might be a great way to get talking to these women and see if they would like a doula at their birth! If you are not sure about who to serve, then start your own support group for pregnant women. We also have a short training called "Bettering Lives of Outstanding Moms" where you can become a leader and start supporting moms in birth (or postpartum). If you want to be this kind of leader, let us know and we will get you set up! You could also start an online group or a meetup.com group. Now that you have some kind of group set up – maybe narrow down your group to be like "First time teen moms" for instance. Decide what you want to make the focus of your group. Once you start having meetings for support, there will probably be a few moms that will "want more" – so these moms are the ones that will end up being your client for doula work! Excellent! Now, you can learn more about business and contracts and such.

Remember it is OK to be picky in the doula business. Moms are going to be picky about who they choose. Be honest with them if you do not have experience. Most moms are willing to try you out! Some may even be looking for a newbie since costs are usually less – but still charge something – do not do births for free – it devalues doula work! My first birth, I got paid $150!

So, we will get you started in business of doula work in this section and show you how to apply more the "Comfort in Birth™" acronym.

Enrichment form for clients

First of all, as you get to know your client mamas, you will want to have an enrichment form for them to fill out if they are going to work with you. This can also be done for virtual clients as well. A form can easily be emailed to the mama. She should fill this out after the free consultation if she is hiring you.

We will put together a sample one for you to look at. The form is meant to gain insight into the mother's likes, dislikes, how many pregnancies she has had before, full viable children, any health issues, etc. This is important for you to know things like this. Also, where does the mother plan to give birth at? Knowing where to go in the middle of the night is good to drive by the place beforehand! If are a virtual doula, you may at least want to know the name of hospital and number just in case you need to reach mother during labor, and you lost contact with her.

Also, we want to make sure the mother knows what your contract covers. We will cover a sample contract in this section.

Question X: What do you think an enrichment form should have in it?

We are not able to put the enrichment form in this book please email instructor for the enrichment form.

***Assignment: Email instructor for enrichment form – have a mother fill out form as a requirement for the class. If you do not have a client yet, you may skip this assignment.

Next, you may want to consider what you will be doing at your prenatals for mothers.

Will you be educating the mother about nutrition if she needs this?

Will you be helping the mother learn about informed consent and hospital procedures? It may vary what you offer at your prenatals. Remember one size does NOT fill all mothers. Having the mother fill out the enrichment form above gives you key ideas and insights to what she may need help with the most. Follow the acronym "Comfort in Birth©" and see where it leads you to the mother's needs for her 2 prenatal visits. If she needs more help, we hope to come up

with a fuller childbirth class method in the future! In the meantime, you may want to add in private childbirth classes if the mother needs extra help. Write down 2 things you will teach a mother for prenatals?

Another thing you need to consider is your birth contract.

We want you to achieve this goal on your own. We will give you some resources to find contracts on the internet. However, I feel that each doula should come up with her own unique style of contract. As of writing this book – all links were working. If one is not just skip to the next resource link!

Resources:

1. Birth contract:
https://www.houseoflukaya.com/pages/birth-doula-service-agreement
2. Postpartum contract example:
https://littlemountaindoula.weebly.com/sample-contract.html
3. Common mistakes of doula contracts:
http://100percentdoula.com/get-clients/4-common-mistakes-of-a-doula-contract
4. Sample Jot Form for doulas:
https://www.jotform.com/form-templates/doula-intake-form
5. Another sample of birth contract:
http://www.enjoybirth.com/doula-agreement.html

*****Challenge***Create your own uniquely "YOU" Doula birth contract. Make sure to read about the tips on what to avoid doing as well (above).**

Submit your birth doula contract for grading to instructor!

Creating Doula Packages!

Creating doula packages can help you obtain a client quicker and faster. Many mamas will just want a "basic" package. However, you can create a medium sized package (a bit more) and then a fancier "extreme" package for your mama client! Giving a mama more than one choice may get you occasional extra funds for your work.

Packages can be created different ways. The simplest way is offering a basic package, possible an "experienced" mama package (which may have less then basic – but the mom would have to go by your criteria of having a baby before and not need extra helping hand for instance), medium package – a few extras; and then like the extreme package where you get all the extras to a mom for more $. Remember to price things that include the postage in it – for instance if you are offering virtual services and sending the mother something in the mail. A small box from the post office that is priority mail is now like $8.30 just to mail the small box – so remember to include postage. Even if you decide not to mail it priority – it is important to know postage estimates or print your own at your house and then drop off! Easy peasy! You may want to offer a special VBAC package for mamas wanting a VBAC birth. Also, get creative with your packages. Having fun names to go with your doula business makes it appealing to clients.

Services Package example:
Package 1: "Baby Steps" Basic support
1 Prenatal Visit
Entire Labour & Birth (90 minutes aftercare)
1 postpartum visit
$600
Package 2: "Honey – I got you covered" Extra support
3 Prenatal Visits

Special Meal Prep Day
Entire Labour & Birth (90 minutes aftercare)
3 Postpartum Visits
$800

Package 3: "Talk Time: Virtual Sessions" – Long Distance Doula Work:
3 Zoom sessions
Unlimited call/text
Birth Support
Detailed Informative Emails
1 Postpartum Zoom Session
$500
Postpartum and the Birth Story!

So, I hope this gives you a good idea on how to set up a package deal for your birth doula services! (Note – exercises below should be turned into instructor if doing for certification).

Fun Exercise: First of all, do you have a business name idea?

If not, there are some "business name generators" – like maybe you have some image ideas of what you want it to be – the business name generator will spit out silly and some good ideas for name. So, think about this first.

Second Exercise: OK, use your "business name idea" (remember this is for fun – you do not have to use this business name if you are unsure still). Use the name you created above for a business name to come up with some package idea names. Also, think of prices that may work in your area. If you are not sure, look up "doulas" in your state to

see what they charge. Make up at least 3 package ideas and write down:

Package A

Package B

Package C

<u>Long distance doula options:</u> This is a new term being used more. Virtual doulas are popping up all over the place. So, what does this mean? How do you support a mother in a long-distance way? Let us explore this:

Long distance doulas can help mothers via phone, Face Time, Skype, or other devices of communication. Good old phone calls or email also works!

Sessions are usually an hour long with the client. Free consultation can still be done via phone or above communication (shorter time frame). The fuller sessions are for paying clients. You can still ask for compensation it is usually less than a regular birth; a price according to what you think your client can pay or afford. Some doulas offer special military discounts or financial need. Make your packaging work for you! We will discuss more about the business of doula later.

Long distance doulas will still prepare a mother for labor and birth. She will help the mother and her partner work together in a better way. If you are not going to be there, then it is key for the partner/husband to be part of this birth experience. The mother may also be choosing her mother to step in for this. So, be clear who will be her "in person" helper at birth. This "in person" helper may be a key person you will communicate with via texting at the birth time.

Sessions will be much like regular prenatals for mothers. Here are some ideas to offer:

a. Birth wishes or birth vision plan

b. Helping mother know about hospital procedures.

c. Helping mom get more familiar with "Birth in Comfort Method©" by helping her relax and go over techniques that can be done over the phone (example: Take Charge routine)

d. Arrange a video or visuals for mom about rebozo.

e. Ask mother what she is fearing and help her with that for instance.

<u>Extra Things to consider for birth:</u>

Making a rice sock for a client can help with pain during labor. Fill a sock with rice and tie it up or sew up the end. Heat it up in microwave for warmth. Put in freezer for cold support.

Making bath bombs for clients is another idea. (This talent is for someone else – I attempted to make bombs and it was a failure -so I do better with sewing things!) I can actually sew rebozos if I have the right fabrics.

We are now planning business master class for all students who trains with us and any other doula; that class will include Business 101, *Doulaing Virtually©* Training plus if you pay extra, you get the certification for that, and so much more! We are so excited to offer this soon. Check Comfort in Birth Website and Catholic Doula Program for details!

Make up a rice sock or bath bomb and submit a picture to us. If you want a bath bomb recipe – let us know and we will find one and share it with you!

Long distance/Virtual Doula Packages:

Long distance doula packages can be different than regular ones. It depends if you are doing more virtual work or not. If you find yourself doing more virtual work, then you may want to create 3 choices for virtual packages.

The package choices can include a zoom call, regular phone call, power point slide presentation or whatever works for you to present your information to the parents. Try to include both mother/father (boyfriend or partner).

As we stated above, we sometimes send out goody bags to moms for virtual services. We usually send this out as a postpartum gift. So, remember to include postage. The lowest goody bag could cost her like $28, second $38, third $48 – something like that. The postage being included.

Why long distance or virtual doula right now? As I write this the terrible "pandemic" is upon us, so the long-distance work is the most way doulas are going right now. Hopefully, there will be some better protocols that will allow doulas to still go to hospitals in the future. More moms are going to homebirth; so, you as a doula should also look into helping moms with homebirth situations as another option!!

Exercise: Think about virtual doula work. Write up a short paragraph or make a pretend package for a virtual doula client. What would it include? Remember to turn in exercises in this chapter to the instructor!

Chapter 19: Heart of the Home Postpartum Visit and more: The Postpartum Visit

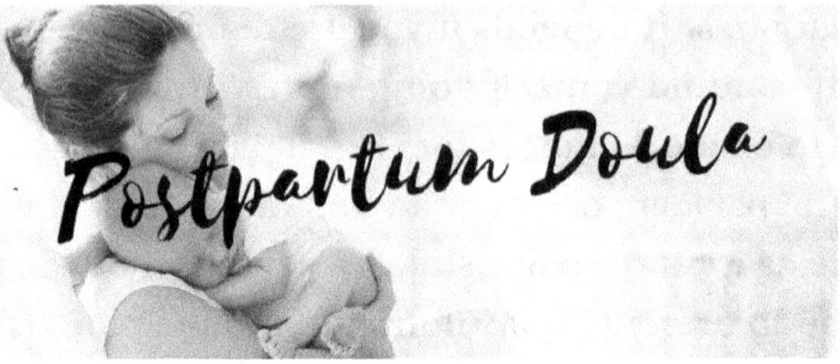

Following up with the mother after birth is important. You get to see the baby one more time. You can choose to offer one visit or 2 postpartum visits. Remember you are not acting as a postpartum doula, but a follow up birth. If the mother seems to need a post-natal doula recommend one or study to become one too!

Birth journal/records: Keeping a birth journal during delivery will be a way to help the mother write down her story about her birth. Perhaps she did not have the birth she wanted. Helping the mother "debrief" about her birth story will make her feel better. Remember if she had a traumatic birth – also discuss this if she is open to it. Are there any medical malpractice from this traumatic birth? If yes, does she want to pursue legal action or not? This is up to her. Presenting her with organizations that work towards helping mothers in this is important. Here is one such organization: http://www.solaceformothers.org/

Question: How to process a birth/traumatic or not that did not go to plan?

A doula becomes part of the mother's birth story. The doula helped the mother with her positioning to comfort measures during the delivery. The doula was there for the mother's emotional needs. Answer below:

1. Explain the value of a birth story and how you can be part of this.

2. What are some things that you can do to fix mistakes, hone your craft, and use to get better?

3. Birth Story – write down a recent birth story that you have gone to *(if not skip).*

Breastfeeding and the new mother:

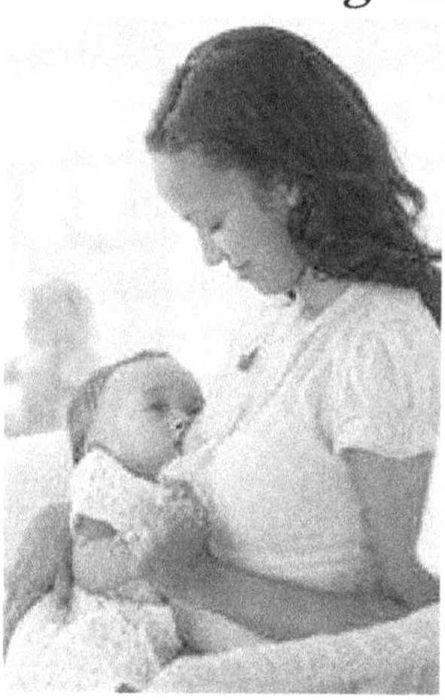

The **new mother** should be encouraged to breastfeed and get this well-established within the first few days.

Some tips for starting up breastfeeding and keep it going:

1. **Make sure the baby is well-latched.** We will link to some videos in our postpartum module. For now, consider looking at a video if you are just reading this booklet for fun.
2. **Make sure the baby is well positioned.** Baby should be skin to skin – belly to mom's belly. No twisting of baby's head or body. This will make a well positioned baby no matter what breastfeeding position you choose.

3. **Make sure mother knows the various breastfeeding positions.** They are cradle, cross-cradle, football hold, laid-back, and side-lying positions. We will cover this more in our "fuller module course". Look up some pictures online if so desired.
4. **First Days:** Make sure mother knows the ins and outs of first few days- the colostrum comes in first and then the "major milk". So, the milk that comes in a few days later may hurt and mom may feel engorged. Having a hand pump or breastfeeding pump to help with this is important.
5. **Feed baby often:** Know the baby will eat every 2-3 hours and most babies do not need a "schedule" this young. Babies need to eat often in order to fill their small tummies!
6. **Pain:** If mother is still having pain or issues from breastfeeding after 2 days, it is important to get help from a lactation counselor sooner than later. Please do contact one for the mother.
7. Ask us about our special M.O.M. advocate class – please email instructor about this. It is a class that teaches you how to run a breastfeeding support group. 😉
8. **Please read a breastfeeding book for review for this course.**
9. Suggested breastfeeding books to review: **The Womanly Art of Breastfeeding** by La Leche League; ***Lactivate!: A User's Guide to Breastfeeding***, ***Breastfeeding Made***

Simple; LATCH-A handbook for breastfeeding with confidence at every stage; ***The Nursing Mother's Companion; Eat to Feed: 80 Nourishing Recipes for Breastfeeding Moms.***

Submit one Breastfeeding book review as part of your certification requirement to catholicdoulaprogram@gmail.com

Postpartum blues and depression:

The mother should seek help if she has lingering symptoms of feeling bad, wanting to hurt herself, anger, anxiety. There are varying degrees of postpartum depression. Sometimes medication is needed. I am currently writing a postpartum book and hope to address more of this in that. If a mother needs help, make sure to discuss it with dad/father and relatives, and suggest mother sees a doctor.

Postpartum home:

A doula should be non-judgmental when visiting mother for your "last time" at your postpartum visit. If you can help a bit when going over for your final visit – ask first. Also, bringing a meal for the mother after birth would probably be something the mother would accept and enjoy. Help arrange community that the mother has access to for future meals. There are Meal Train, Care Calendar, and others that help arrange meals for those in need. Usually, a church will help with this. If the person is not connected with a church, you may ask the mother if you can arrange for your church or community center to set up something. Gift cards for meals is also a wonderful idea. I remember obtaining some pizza gift cards and another one for a nice restaurant. Well, I was able to use the cards like a couple months or so after I had the baby. I kind of felt guilty, but then figured it was a nice treat not to have to cook.

Read some further books about postpartum as one of your book reviews: "The First Forty days" is one of my favorite ones. Just the pictures that pop and make you go "wow". The recipes and more.

Recommended reading for postpartum:

- **The Postpartum Depression Workbook: Strategies to Overcome Negative Thoughts, Calm Stress, and Improve Your Mood**
- **This Isn't What I Expected: Overcoming Postpartum Depression**
- **The Fourth Trimester: A Postpartum Guide to Healing Your Body, Balancing Your Emotions, and Restoring Your Vitality**
- **Postpartum depression and anxiety: A self-help guide for mothers**
- **The Postpartum Husband: Practical Solutions for living with Postpartum Depression**
- **Creating Postpartum Wellness by Laura Rude**
- **A Catholic Postpartum by Julie Larsen**

*****Required: Read one postpartum depression book or self-help book listed above and submit review to instructor.**

Some other tips to consider:

If dad is available after birth and mother is suffering from depression; get him in on helping out more and doing things around the house. See if dad can take extra time off from his work if possible!

Make a dad to do list. If a relative can come help – make the relative a to do list.

If you are a doula and take the Nutritional doula class then you will have more skills on helping moms cook and prepare their meals. You may even want to start your own meal service for postpartum mothers!

Thanking your client!

Remember to send a little thank you card or small gift to your client for being their doula. If you want to create a package with a postpartum item in it – make sure to charge extra for this postpartum package! They will thank you later for doing so! You are a powerful doula and you helped this mother; make sure she will want to hire you again! Repeat clients of the same mother is possible! Write down a way you would like to thank your mother client!

Assignment for this section: Write down how you will conduct your postpartum visit, what you will do in it, and any postpartum gift you might send if doing a virtual doula option (or also you can give a gift if in person doula). Submit to instructor.

Chapter 20: The Holistic/Whole doula[lxxvii]:

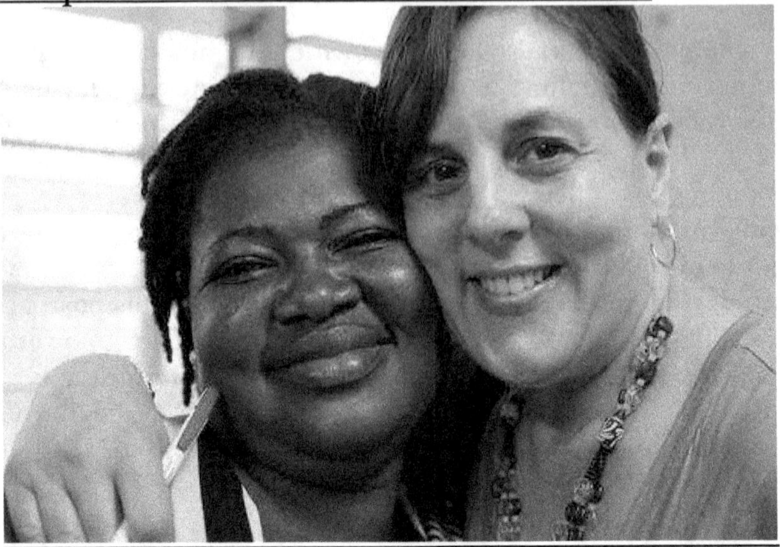

What does "whole doula" mean? As a doula we are holistic and also look at the mother as a "whole person".

What do we mean by the "whole doula?" I wanted to add on this little bit of extra information before going on to certification.

The Whole doula means that we give our hands, hearts, minds, and body to help the mothers we serve. If you are Christian, you do this through Jesus Christ as well. The whole doula also knows how to stop and take care of oneself as well.

This concept is something we must consider; if we get overwhelmed with clients and do not stop to care for ourselves then we are going to get burn out. I know that a beginning doula may not see themselves getting burned out or tired of this beautiful work of seeing and helping babies come into the world, but it can happen to a doula or midwife.

One way to prevent burnout is to have a backup doula. If a birth looks like it is going to be long and you know you need a break, call in the back up for the first portion of the longer part of labor and be nearby to pick up the phone and know when the labor is getting to the point of pushing. Your backup should be experienced enough to know when to call you back into the birth. Then, you can go up to the hospital or home (depending on the location of birth) and finish up the birth time with your client.

This is a needed time to care for oneself is also after a birth. If you are overbooked and have 2-3 births together then you may not be able to "come up for air" or "take a break". Believe me when I say you would be better off giving one of these births on your list to another doula – perhaps one that is just starting up. So, if you are a doula who is just starting up, talk to local doulas and ask to be their backup. You may find that this doula "gifts you" a client because she is too busy!

Meeting with clients as a "whole doula". When you meet a client for the first time, be yourself. If they like you, they will hire you, and if not, they will not. It is as simple as that. Do not take it personally. However, also what if you are hired and you don't feel a connection? Then, you may want to politely give them a refund and ask them to find another doula. This is okay as well. It is better to mesh well at the beginning and to be disturbed at the end as to why you worked with the mother.

A whole doula is also holistic and wants to be helpful for mothers. There are a lot of hours and stamina for doula work. If you have some weaknesses, you may want to consider this before jumping in as a doula! Being an emotional doula is ok as long as you can keep them in check when working with clients. Everyone can get emotional once in a while. If something happens, that you regret saying – be apologetic –

but not too much. Admit your mistake and do not be argumentative. It will not get you good reviews.

Another thing to consider, if you are working late at night, instead of driving to a birth, you may want to get a ride over (maybe hubby drop you off) and then get Uber or something like that to pick you up and drop you back off home. This helps because you won't have to worry about driving when tired!

Here are some other questions to consider that you can fill out and write down to see if this helps you with finding and keeping clients:

What type of clients attract you? Do you accept all clients that come to you? There is not right or wrong answer. Who's your idea client and why?

Write down a name of a person who can be your "backup" doula?

Remember our earlier section about doula packages – what can you offer that is unique to make your package stand out?

Do you have a website yet? What's your business name?

Write down all of above and send answers to instructor if taking class for grading.

In conclusion, we hope that this newly improved version of Comfort in Birth Method will help you become the best doula practitioner out there for mothers.

Remember to look for the certification checklist at the end of this book if you are taking this as class credit – you will need to finish all assignments, quizzes and ask for any missing quizzes that are not in this book. Remember to do skill assignments such as rebozo and comfort techniques. Thank you.

We also are adding in a couple of birth stories.

If you are a mother and have decided to try out our method, we would love to hear about your successful birth using the *Comfort in Birth Method* technique. Please email author at catholicdoulaprogram@gmail.com

Also, note there were some quizzes not included in this book, please email instructor for any quizzes missing and we will send them to you. The anatomy of birth section will need to be also emailed to you the labeling exercise! This is for registered students only through: Catholic Doula Program or Fruit of Thy Womb doula courses. https://fruitofthywombdoula.weebly.com

**Certification requirements are on page 262. Thank you.

Birth Story Appendix A: Amanda's story:

"My first baby was an unexpected delivery. I was expecting my baby to come around October 8th, but that day came and went without any labor pains. I did have Braxton-Hicks contractions on a nightly basis. It seemed like my little one was wanting to practice every time I tried to go to sleep. Anyway, fast forward to 41 weeks, I started having some GI distress cramping and bloating and just feeling out of sorts. It started at 4 am on October 15th. I woke up my husband complaining of the GI distress. He helped me into the bathroom a few times. I managed to get maybe an hour or two of sleep before the GI stuff acted up again. I started seeing blood in my poop and started getting frightened. My husband decided to call a doctor up and ask about it. I wanted to go straight to the ER. The doctor suggested timing the contractions or spams I was having. My husband noticed a rhythm to them. The doctor said, 'she sounds like she's in labor – call an ambulance if she cannot move.' So, my husband decided to call an ambulance team and they came over to the house. It took me some time to go from the mode of 'I am in GI stress' to 'we are having a baby.' However, my husband remembered reading about the Comfort in Birth Method book and C stands for Calm. He grabbed my hand and held it while we waited for the ambulance and said, 'C is for calm – Christ is in this calm and you can get this baby to come on down'. My husband's whispers really helped me feel better even though the contractions felt weird and really low in my abdomen. The ER crew arrived quickly and by the time they arrived the baby's head was already starting to come out. My husband said as I was pushing baby out 'O is for Open – remember to relax as you open up for baby'. I smiled and did one last push and baby came out; the ER tech handed me the baby. My husband said, 'It's a girl.' I smiled. Well, she definitely came as a surprise delivery! The ER person asked, 'What are you going to name her?' I replied, 'M for Mariana.' My husband smiled and nodded in agreement. I was also able to push out the placenta at home and basically complete the whole birth at home. We did agree to go to hospital after to make sure baby and I were okay. Everyone was okay. I decided to stay overnight, and we both came home the next day."[lxxviii]

Second Birth Story: Maria's Birth Story: "My labor started at 2 am in the morning. My water broke. My contractions started right away. I called my midwife up and she helped me with breathing. I decided to try getting into a shower to help relieve my contraction pain and relax. I also was thinking 'C for comfort' as I really felt more comfortable in the shower. My midwife said she would come over when things were speeding up more. I decided to try to go back to sleep. I woke up at 8 am and labor started to intensify. I called my midwife, and she came right over. My midwife's name was Katherine or Katy. Katy had an assistant named Beth. They asked me if I still wanted a waterbirth. I thought my contractions were coming too fast, so I decided to decline it right then. I felt like this baby was going to be here quickly. We decided to set up towels and pads on the bed. I just felt like 'giving birth on land' is going to be better for this baby. During my wait for the baby to come, I kind of went into like a 'M for Meditation' during labor. I kept concentrating on breathing and the surges. I felt like I was in a rhythm. My husband was there supporting me throughout the whole way. At one point, I felt like I needed to poop, my midwife figured it was probably pushing time. She checked me and said I was completely dilated, and it was time to start pushing. I got on the bed, and I started to push. It took a few pushes, and my baby came out. My midwife unwrapped the cord wrapped around the baby's neck. My husband announced, 'It's a boy!' I smiled. My midwife said, 'What are you going to name him?' I smiled and said Gabriel is his name. We were so happy with our home birth!"[lxxix]

Appendix B: Birth Bag Project – for Doulas: We may have mentioned this in the book, but this is for you to consider as a project.

Create a birth bag that you would like to use for your doula services. Please purchase items you want to use in it: massage tool, rebozo shawl, ice pack or make a rice sock, etc. Take a picture of your birth bag project and this can count towards your community project or final project assignment. Count how many hours you took to put together your bag. (For instance – 2 hours).

Appendix C: Finding Doula Client Tips: First of all, a lot of mothers still do not know what doulas are or what we do. So, we suggest hosting a few "what is a doula" seminars or workshops in your area. This can be done at a library since it is a free event. It could be done at a church or recreation center. Ask around where you can offer such free events. You might be able to do it at a chiropractic office for instance. Remember to advertise your event – maybe put an ad in the newspaper or digital news service or the library may advertise it for you as well.

Second idea, start a mothering group. Learn about our B.L.O.O.M. program. I believe I am going to make a B.L.O.O.M. training manual up soon, so we can make it a consistent training for leaders. As a "Bettering Lives of Outstanding Moms" leader you will be able to work with pregnant or postpartum mothers. In the meantime, email the instructor if you want more information about this. You can also create your own style group for this.

Third, start your own mother group on Facebook/online. This is another way to connect with mothers in your area.

Fourth, make sure you contact other "healers" in your area – chiropractors, doctors, massage therapists, etc. Get to know them. Add these people to your resource list and see if they are willing to add you back. Doctors like OB/gyns – you can write them a letter of introduction and send that to them. See what places will allow you to put your business card out.

Fifth, Contact boutiques, shops that sell baby clothes, etc. This might also be a place where you can host a "What is a doula" event.

Lastly, social media pages and such are always a good idea too! Need more help please read *Doing Business the Doula Way book.*

***Certification Checklist:

To become fully certified in our Comfort in Birth Method class – if doing this class as "Comfort in Birth Method" you will need to submit a doula course mentorship fee payment and certification fee – see what that is at Fruit of Thy Womb Doula https://fruitofthywombdoula.weebly.com

Comfort in Birth™ Doula Certification Checklist:

1. Read through "The Comfort in Birth™ Book"
2. Do all the exercises in this manual. If you are a previous trained doula; please ask us for exceptions.
3. Make a 20-resource list for mothers – you may have started this with one of the case studies in the book.
4. Make up a website for your doula business – you will include the 20-resource list in it and any other items you wish to add.
5. Write 5 book reviews –they should cover the following topics: a) any pregnancy book, b) any nutrition and pregnancy or challenges of birth, c) breastfeeding, d) postpartum depression, e) VBAC book review.
6. Attend a childbirth class online or in person. If you need an online class, we offer a St. Zélie or St. Gianna childbirth class for parents – you can review a module or two from that class and we will count it. If you prefer a non-denominational style class – let us know and we will help you find something.

7. Interview 3 mothers about their birth experiences. Please reference this manual – One interview can be about emotions and birth for instance.

8. Please do the Royal Rebozo way skills listed in this manual and turn it in for grading. If you want full Level A and B certificates – you need to take our live or pre-recorded class to receive that certification – we will offer a discount to all students to view those materials. (It is optional for you to receive that certification).

10. Take your final exam. Pass with at least 75 percent – you have the option to take it again. We allow open book study for the exam. Email instructor for final exam. Catholic Doula students do community project in lieu of final exam.

11. Final Project Options: Attend ONE Birth, Document hours working with a mother 10-20 hours, Nutritional Doula with detailed food diary, Contact teacher with your own ideas or Complete the PEACE project (at appendix area) with a mother (via email if necessary).

If this project is too complicated - you can also do the enrichment form using the words "Comfort in Birth" acronym with a mother (if actually going to a birth – this would probably work better for you).

We are also open to any other ideas for a final project. The final project just needs to have at least 2-4 hours of documented time spent on it! Thank you so much!

Appendix F – Food Diary:

Food Diary Form:

Food Diary Day:	Protein	Vegetables	Grains	Dairy/sweet
Day 1				
Day 2				
Day 3				
Day 4				
Day 5				
Day 6				
Day 7				

Name three things the mother needs to change in her diary in order to have healthier foods (unless she is eating "healthy" already).

Submit to instructor diary and suggestions.

<u>Interview questions for asking mothers about birth. (Remember to do 3 times)</u>

1. Your name:
2. Baby name (optional):
3. When was the baby born? How much did baby weigh?
4. Did you have a c-section, epidural, natural birth?
5. Tell us about the emotions of this birth:
6. Tell us about if you had any person "doula" for you (relative or friend or hired a doula? Husband?)
7. How did your support person help you during your delivery?
8. How did your support person help BEFORE delivery?
9. How did your support person help AFTER delivery?
10. What is one thing you would change about your birth experience or story?
11. Share your birth story in full (if so desired).
12. If you did not know about doulas, would you have "hired one" if money was not an object (if that is) for your birth? Would you consider having one for your next baby?
13. Did you ever hear of Comfort in Birth Method or read the book?

Feel free to ask other questions if so desired.

<u>Book Review Form:</u> (Remember to submit 5 book reviews if taking for Comfort in Birth Student Program if taking for Catholic Doula Program – 3-4 book reviews will be required).

Student:

Date:

Book:

Author:

How would you rate the book 1-10 (1 poor - 10 best)

Would you encourage others to read? If so, who?

What are a few things you learned?

What did you disagree with?

Did you take notes to study?

Childbirth class attendance form (or breastfeeding class)
Your name (Julie) attended the childbirth or breastfeeding class – Online or in person (circle one)
On the date of __________________________________.
Instructor's name____.
Please submit it to us.
If you would like you can take a class from www.catholicdoula.com ask about the parent childbirth class offerings.

Appendix R: Other Resources:

Yiska Obadia: http://www.yiskaobadia.com/workshops
Betsy Schwartz: www.birthintheknow.com
Maha Al Musa: www.mahalamusa.com – Belly Dance for Birth© Embody Birth© Founder
Noeleen Lang: www.birthbasics.com
Catholic Doula Program: http://catholicdoula.com
Academy of Natural Birth: http://academyofnaturalbirth.weebly.com
Find a Catholic doula: http://findacatholicdoula.weebly.com
Breastfeeding University – become a Peer Counselor and more: http://uobreast.weebly.com

Author bibliography:

Julie Larsen is the founder of Comfort in Birth Method. Her credentials include studying with Birth Arts International in 2010-2011. She received full certification for Childbirth Education from them. She

also received a Hypno-Doula certificate from HypnoBabies in 2011. She trained with Madriella Network in 2014 and 2017 (renewed). She is also the founder of Catholic Doula Program – a spiritual training program. She took other classes from Gena Kirby in 2012 (rebozo), Polly Perez (2013), Intuitive Childbirth Postpartum (2015), H.E.R.B.A.L. Breastfeeding course (2019).

<u>Appendix P: PEACE Project:</u>

P.E.A.C.E. Birth Project – Extra Section (This is for your final project or you can choose another final project).

We are going to cover this acronym to help you become a better Comfort in Birth Practitioner!

P = Positive Birth and Peaceful Birth

E = Emotions at Birth (we already covered some)

A = Active Birth; Allowing God in the birth room (if Christian)

C = Comfort in Birth Method™ and having a Calm birth!

E = Enjoy Birth and Entering Postpartum!

We want you to find a mother to work with for this project. You may consider this a "final project" to help you establish your birth knowledge better.

P for Positive:

1. What is a positive birth? Definition from Positive Birth Movement website is this: "A positive birth means a birth in which a woman feels she has freedom of choice, access to accurate information, and that she is in control, powerful and respected." Source: https://www.positivebirthmovement.org

We think a positive birth means:
Women are where they want to be
Choices are informed by reality not fear
Women are listened to and treated with respect and dignity
Mothers are empowered and enriched
Memories are warm and proud

P for positive: Assignment for your community project blog/website: Find a birth story online or perhaps interview a mother in your community about her birth experience. Find a mother who can give you a positive or peaceful birth story (should be at least no C-section for this one– prefer a natural birth story if possible). Have her tell her story and you can ask a few questions. Put her story and answers to the questions on your community project blog/website. Also, submit the interview story for grading.

E for Emotions and Emotional Dystocia:

We covered a lot about emotions in an earlier chapter – feel free to go back and read through that. The "Letting go of Fears" assignment can also be used as part of this section. So, if you have not done that assignment please do so now with a pregnant mother.

What is emotional dystocia? This can happen in labor when a certain emotion might come up from the mother's past and make it difficult for her to continue labor. It could be a bad memory, abusive memory, etc. If the mother had previous "sexual abuse" or "rape" then this might be a time to try to get the mom through this part of labor. There is a book titled "Survivor's Give Birth" – we highly recommend working with a mother that has suffered this in the past. The bad memory could be of a baby that was miscarried. In that case, you may want to know more about bereavement issues. I wrote a book titled "Hope Through Sorrow" – this is a Catholic booklet – but can be helpful if mom is open to Christian reading material. She may want to read "Joy at the End of the Rainbow: A Guide for Pregnancy After Loss."

Here are some resource websites for mothers who may have emotional dystocia during labor and some tips to follow:

https://healingmidwifery.blogspot.com/2009/01/what-is-emotional-dystocia-during-labor.html

This article covers three types of dystocia: https://vital-wellbeing.com/birth-dystocia-what-you-need-to-know / (Physical, Emotional and Lactogenic (things just slow down on purpose). Something from this article might be on final exam.

https://www.romper.com/p/emotional-dystocia-is-something-all-moms-to-be-need-to-know-heres-why-8770360

Assignment for "E" emotions and dystocia: Interview a mother about her birth experience (try to find a mother that had emotional time or dystocia that is willing to share her experience). Find out what happened during her birth? What emotions was she feeling? Did she know why this happened? Ask her to share anything that is relevant to this topic. Turn in for grading. (If you cannot find someone – we will assign something else).

<u>A for Active Birth; Allowing God into the Birth Room</u>

Active Birth: Active birth we have kind of covered some of this topic when we talked about birthing upright. So, I invite you to ask the mother you are working with to consider birthing more in an upright position if she can figure this out – maybe being on a birthstool or in the tub in water with a person holding her up.

Allowing God into the Birth Room: Many of you may not be Christian – but if you are this is a time to think about allowing God into the Birth room. What does that mean exactly? It can be simple as listening to his prompts through others or the mother. If we are supporting the mother and she says something like "This just does not feel right – can we pray?" Then do that! It can be that the mother may have intuition to do something different. For example: "My body is telling me to try that maneuver where I go upside down to re-position the baby." Then, the mother should be allowed to follow her intuition. Another way of allowing God into the birth room is through prayer. The mother may have a form of prayer she prefers. Since I tend to work with Catholic mothers: The Rosary is a form of prayer that helps them. A Christian mother may want to recite "Jesus Mercy" several times. Ask the mother if she has prayers that lift her up. Another way is having an affirmation card with a prayer on it.

<u>Assignment:</u> Make an affirmation card up that is prayerful for a mother. Or Ask a mother if she ever felt "intuition" during birth and where did this prompting lead her for her baby's delivery?

Extra Credit: Interview a mom about a "spiritual" experience that she may have had during labor and birth. Submit to instructor.

C for Comfort in Birth Method (or Calm Birth):

C = Calm: How can we help a mother stay calm and cool and collective during birth? If you are a more seasoned doula, you probably been to many births where the mother is crying out in anguish or something like that. Or perhaps you have only seen the TV version of birth. So, for this exercise – find a calm birth video to watch!

Here are a couple of video links: HypnoBirthing:
https://www.youtube.com/watch?v=B3t6av4rARg

Natural birth at a birth center:
https://www.youtube.com/watch?v=qsJWGK5LOdo

Michelle's birth story:
https://www.youtube.com/watch?v=ovI0FvO4t_o

Another birth:
https://www.youtube.com/watch?v=TnN6Ohte9dA

O = Opening up the Body! This can be done by positions and getting on a birth ball. Opening up also can be done on the facial level. The lips are kind of a gateway to the vagina! Make sure mom's lips are not chapped. Make sure mom keeps her mouth relaxed. Have mom practice saying "o" or "open" if she is feeling stuck! (Try this tip at the next birth you attend!)

M = Meditation/Mother! The mother needs to relax during birth and one way is meditation. If the mother is religious, she may have a preferred way to meditate. Also, the mother could focus on an image during this time of meditation. For instance: Maria is Catholic and wanted to focus on the image of Mary Mother Guadalupe and pray or meditate on the image. (Try this tip at the next birth you go to). Write down ways you like to meditate.

F = Letting go of Fears/Do not be afraid of failure. A mother may have fears as described previously – if a mother needs to – please have her do the "Letting go of fears" exercise described in previous chapter. Another thing it is okay for the mother to "seem to fail". If the birth ends up needing an epidural or C-section – this is still a birth that is successful. Let the mother know that she may have emotions of not getting the natural birth she wanted – but she is not a failure – she had a beautiful birth. Look at the positive aspects of birth.

F can also stand for Fathers at the birth! Fathers should be included as much as possible for they are there to help the mother. Include dad in helping the mother with any tool or technique you have to offer. If you are using a massage tool on the mother, ask the dad if he would like to do this instead. Make sure dad gets to cut that cord! You may want to read "Fathers at Birth" by Rose St. John to get more ideas on helping fathers.

Assignment: Research fathers at birth – find an article or read a book. Write 3 things you learned about fathers and birth. If you read a book it can count for one of your 3 book reviews. Or you can interview a dad!

O = Oxytocin: Using as much natural oxytocin during delivery. Oxytocin is known as the "love hormone" and this hormone naturally occurs during childbirth and "labor land" time. Oxytocin naturally helps with pain and usually a mother will have less pain. A Pitocin delivery is the synthetic oxytocin. So, if a mother is choosing Pitocin – remind her that this is not natural and she may have some reactions to the drug. However, we are here to support the mother's choices in labor and delivery as well. One thing a mother can try is using a breast pump and pumping her milk (yep) before baby comes. This pumping can help bring on a better labor pattern if she needs labor to start and has not started yet. (For instance if her water broke, etc.) So, suggest using the breast pump for a mother if she needs the "love hormone" during birth!

R = Relaxation! The mother needs to be reminded to relax. Also, it can stand for Relaxation, Rhythm, and Ritual. Ask the mother if she desires any particular ritual at her birth time? Write this down if working with a mother for a grade.

T= Tools for birth. These items can be massage tool, rebozo, etc.

Write down one tool you want to use for the births you attend – submit for grade.

BIRTH – the rest of the acronym we will summarize briefly:

B for buoyancy – if the mother is open to a water birth – then help her with this. Also, this can also mean having a bath for the baby after birth. Michael Odent uses baths for babies after birth. Suggest a bath for baby after birth to a mother.

I is for Intuition and Imagination! Let the mother use her intuition and imagination during labor – getting her relaxing to a hypnobirthing CD for instance can help.

R for Rhythm and Ritual – Add that to your resource list a person that may do a particular ritual for parents (like naming a child, baptisms, etc.)

T for Time for Baby – Baby will come when he/she wants to come – being patient is always important as a doula. Impatience shows lack of character. Remember to be positive as you wait for baby to arrive. When baby arrives – make sure mother gets to hold baby first, etc. before you ask to hold the baby (if mom allows this).

H for Healing/Help: Birth can be healing for mothers. H for help shows that you as a doula know when to come in and help and know when to stay back and observe. Be the more observant doula if possible. Only offer a helping hand if requested!

Birth Bag assignment: Now, that you have some more ideas on how to use the Comfort in Birth method with our PEACE Project – make a Birth bag that you will put all your wonderful "goodies" in as a doula. Submit a picture of your bag and list of items inside the bag! (If you have not done so already).

E is for Entering Postpartum

Now that the mother has her baby. She is now officially postpartum mother! She has wonderful "energy" immediately after birth. However, this "high" may go away in a few days a week or two. She may find herself in a time of depression. There is natural "baby blues" that should only last a week or so. If she is getting bad thoughts and unusual symptoms – like crying all the time, etc. Then she should seek a doctor's help for her symptoms of depression. It is always better to seek this help sooner than later.

Book recommends: "A Catholic Postpartum" by Julie Larsen (me) is a book I wrote specifically for Catholic mothers; but I think a Christian mother would benefit from reading the book. "Creating Postpartum Wellness" by Laura Rude is another book we recommend for mothers to read.

Assignment: Find an article about postpartum blues vs. depression – write a short summary of this article to turn in for grade! Find a doctor that helps mothers with depression. Add him to your resource list for mothers.

End Notes: Pictures that do not have credits are unknown or creative commons. Thank you.

---

[i] https://pixabay.com/photos/business-women-woman-work-young-3685133/

[ii] This Photo by Unknown Author is licensed under CC BY-NC-ND

[iii] Rosa birth story given permission to share.

[iv] This Photo by Unknown Author is licensed under CC BY-NC-ND

[v] https://www.mexican-clothing-co.com/mexican-rebozo.html
https://www.mexican-clothing-co.com/mexican-rebozo.html

[vi] This Photo by Unknown Author is licensed under CC BY-SA

[vii] same as above

[viii] article here if you would like to read it: https://www.history.com/news/royal-birth-traditions-marie-antoinette-meghan-markle

[ix] (https://www.whattoexpect.com/pregnancy/labor-and-delivery/history-of-childbirth/)

[x] If you would like to read more about the history of granny midwives go here: https://www.lamaze.org/Connecting-the-Dots/black-history-month-the-importance-of-black-midwives-then-now-and-tomorrow-1)

[xi] (Source: https://www.mother.ly/life/pregnancy-tests-have-existed-since-1350-bcand-6-other-insane-facts-on-the-history-of-childbirth#)

[xii] Same source as above (Motherly article)

[xiii] Same source – Motherly article.
[xiv] (Another source: https://www.bellybelly.com.au/birth/twilight-sleep)
[xv] (Source: https://www.llli.org/about/history)
[xvi] https://doulatrainingsinternational.com/brief-history-black-midwifery-us/
[xvii] https://www.nursing-midwifery.tcd.ie/postgraduate/assets/img/hdip2.jpg
[xviii] https://wellwisp.com/how-is-oxytocin-released/
[xix] Source: https://wellwisp.com/how-is-oxytocin-released/
[xx] Source: Ana Pichard – unsplash.com
[xxi] Picture Credit: Mel Elis@ unsplash.com
[xxii] Picture credit: Jonathan Borba @ unsplash.com
[xxiii] Midwifery Today Article – sorry don't know exact one.
[xxiv] This Photo by Unknown Author is licensed under CC BY-NC-ND
[xxv] Nine Golden Months pg. 150
[xxvi] https://online.maryville.edu/blog/types-of-listening/
[xxvii] https://blog.tcea.org/eight-tips-practicing-active-listening-classroom/
[xxviii] Same above article.
[xxix] https://www.verywellhealth.com/female-body-diagram-5209032
[xxx] https://www.healthline.com/health/types-of-pelvis
[xxxi] https://www.verywellhealth.com/female-body-diagram-5209032
[xxxii] Same as above.
[xxxiii] https://www.healthline.com/health/types-of-pelvis
[xxxiv] https://www.healthline.com/health/types-of-pelvis
[xxxv] https://my.clevelandclinic.org/health/body/22467-uterus
[xxxvi] https://omahabirthandbabies.com/seven-cardinal-movements-for-birth/
[xxxvii] https://omahabirthandbabies.com/seven-cardinal-movements-for-birth/
[xxxviii] https://www.lifewithgremlins.com/pregnancy-and-labor-related-terms-simplified/
[xxxix] https://www.lifewithgremlins.com/pregnancy-and-labor-related-terms-simplified/
[xl] https://www.lifewithgremlins.com/pregnancy-and-labor-related-terms-simplified/
[xli] https://www.lifewithgremlins.com/pregnancy-and-labor-related-terms-simplified/
[xlii] https://www.lifewithgremlins.com/pregnancy-and-labor-related-terms-simplified/
[xliii] https://www.lifewithgremlins.com/pregnancy-and-labor-related-terms-simplified/
[xliv] (Birth Conspiracy pg. 133)
[xlv] Pg. 136 Birth Conspiracy.
[xlvi] http://wisewomanwayofbirth.com/tag/gestational-diabetes/
[xlvii] http://wisewomanwayofbirth.com/tag/gestational-diabetes /
[xlviii] https://www.hyperemesis.org/about-hyperemesis-gravidarum
[xlix] https://www.bellybelly.com.au/birth/what-is-a-cervical-lip-how-can-it-hijack-your-birth/
[l] https://www.thebump.com/a/birthing-positions - picture reference https://www.bellybelly.com.au/birth/what-is-a-cervical-lip-how-can-it-hijack-your-birth/
[li] Unsplash photo credit
[lii] Creative commons picture
[liii] Picture credit: bich-ngoc-le-tslOpGXKj-c-unsplash.jpg
[liv] (Resource: Birth Conspiracy Book Chapter 16)
[lv] Creative Commons Picture. This Photo by Unknown Author is licensed under CC BY-NC-ND
[lvi] Pg. 170 *The Birth Conspiracy* book.
[lvii] (Quote from Modern Reflexology article). Modern Reflexology: https://www.modernreflexology.com/acupressure-points-for-easing-labor-pains/
[lviii] Mama Natural: https://www.mamanatural.com/how-to-do-acupressure-when-youre-in-labor/
[lix] This Photo by Unknown Author is licensed under CC BY

[lx] Source: http://www.herbnclay.com/blog/calcium-bentonite-clay-help-healthy-pregnancy/

[lxi] (Source: https://www.havening.org/about-havening/faqs)

[lxii] https://i.pinimg.com/originals/1b/12/dc/1b12dce1883aebb3a1af5d456035283e.jpg

[lxiii] (Source: Herbal Healing for Women by Rosemary Gladstar pg. 176).

[lxiv] Source: Herbal Healing for Women by Rosemary Gladstar pg. 176). And for the other herbs listed.

[lxv] (Source is Herbal Healing for Women by Rosemary Gladstar pg. 177-178)

[lxvi] (Source: Herbal Healing for Women by Rosemary Gladstar – pg. 179)

[lxvii] (pg. 180 above source).

[lxviii] Wikipedia https://en.wikipedia.org/wiki/Lunge_%28exercise%29

[lxix] https://www.spinningbabies.com/pregnancy-birth/techniques/other-techniques/lunge/

[lxx] IBID.

[lxxi] IBID.

[lxxii] (The Birth Partner, Simkin, pg.115)

[lxxiii] https://americanpregnancy.org/healthy-pregnancy/pregnancy-complications/placenta-previa-923/

[lxxiv] This Photo by Unknown Author is licensed under CC BY-ND Creative Commons.

[lxxv] https://www.mamanatural.com/padsicles/

[lxxvi] (Picture – a student Laura with her friend trying out the dangle pose).

[lxxvii] This Photo by Unknown Author is licensed under CC BY-NC-ND

[lxxviii] Used with permission from Amanda S. Birth Story.

[lxxix] Used with permission from Mariana R. Birth Story.